Patients' Rights and Doctors' Wrongs® - Secrets to a Safer Pregnancy and Childbirth

Patients' Rights and Doctors' Wrongs® - Secrets to a Safer Pregnancy and Childbirth

Howard A. Janet, Esq. & Giles H. Manley, MD, JD

ISBN-10: 1512279951
ISBN-13: 9781512279955

DEDICATIONS

This book is dedicated to the many private practice and university-affiliated obstetricians who have stood with me to help families harmed by substandard care delivered during pregnancy and childbirth. I learned so much from them, including the importance of encouraging and enabling expectant mothers to be informed, proactive participants in their obstetrical care.

—*Howard A. Janet, Esq.*

This book is dedicated to the thousands of expectant mothers who afforded me the privilege of caring for them. They gladly embraced my philosophy that informed and inquisitive patients help doctors provide optimal care. Their questions helped me to be a better doctor.

—*Giles H. Manley, MD, JD*

Table of Contents

PART I

Introduction

Samantha's Story

Samantha is beginning to worry. She's been awake for well over an hour, but hasn't felt her baby move. Ordinarily, she feels him move four to five times an hour in the mornings. Samantha is glad she is to see her obstetrician (OB) today for a regularly scheduled appointment. *It's probably nothing,* she thinks. *The baby's just sleeping. I'm getting all worked up over nothing.* But she continues to have doubts, as any expectant mother would. She craves her doctor's assurance that her baby is well.

Samantha is thirty-eight weeks pregnant. She has diabetes, so her pregnancy is considered high-risk. Taking appropriate precautions, Samantha decided to entrust her care and that of her baby, whom she has already named Robert, to an obstetrical group that includes a specialist in high-risk pregnancy known as a *maternal fetal specialist*. The specialist managing her care recommended that Samantha undergo an elective C-section when it's time for delivery. She agreed and is scheduled for surgery in two weeks.

The reason for Samantha's appointment this morning is to perform a non-stress test (NST), a simple, non-invasive test performed in pregnancies after the twenty-eighth week to assess the baby's well-being. The test is so-named because it puts no stress on the fetus. The test involves attaching one belt to the mother's abdomen to measure fetal heart rate and another belt to measure contractions. Movement, heart rate and reactivity of heart rate to movement are measured for twenty to thirty minutes.

Samantha's doctor has instructed her to eat regularly, so before heading out the door, she takes time to eat a light breakfast of toast with sugar-free strawberry jelly, followed by a glass of skim milk. With a little food in her tummy, she feels better physically and mentally. Her mood improves. *Everything has been going just as it should,* she thinks. *My baby has been right on track every time I've seen the doctor. There's no reason to think that's changed.*

But she's still not able to shake those nagging worries. The baby is still. No little elbows nudging her. No kicks, rolls, or wiggles. Samantha rushes to her appointment and tells her doctor about the baby's lack of movement as soon as she arrives.

At this stage of pregnancy, establishing the presence of fetal movement is essential. A baby that exhibits adequate fetal movement and a normal heart rate is classified as *reactive*, with adequate blood flow (and oxygen) to the fetus. That is what everyone wants. A *non-reactive* result requires additional testing to determine whether the result is due to poor oxygenation or there are other reasons for fetal non-reactivity.

Samantha's high-risk obstetrician conducts electronic fetal heart monitoring (EFM), which can detect fetal movement that is imperceptible to the mother. A reactive baby's heart rate should speed up or accelerate when fetal movement occurs. In Samantha's case, no accelerations are detected during twenty minutes of EFM. The OB is concerned, but it is possible the baby is just sleeping. He maintains a poker face, tells Samantha there is no reason for alarm, and suggests performing a biophysical profile (BPP).

Using ultrasound equipment, the OB begins the BPP procedure, which uses sound to stimulate fetal movement. When he presses a buzzer, the noise travels through the amniotic fluid, but produces no fetal movement. That's not good news. The OB stops the biophysical profile in its tracks.

He tells Samantha it's time for her baby to be delivered, and immediately sends her to the hospital, which is just a short wheelchair ride away. A nurse alerts the hospital that the patient is on her way over for a C-section. The referring OB writes a note explaining why Samantha is being sent for delivery at this time, and sends it with her to the hospital. He expects the C-section to be performed without delay unless further testing upon arrival at the hospital demonstrates the baby's condition has significantly improved.

By the time she reaches the hospital, Samantha is extremely alarmed. *I thought the doctor would say everything was fine. Something must be terribly wrong. Oh, God, please let my baby be all right!*

A nurse in the labor-and-delivery suite evaluates Samantha and her baby upon admission. Despite the phone call from the high-risk OB's nurse and the explanatory entry in Samantha's chart, the nurse writes in the hospital chart that Samantha has presented for an elective C-section.

A resident physician in his early years of training to become a specialist in obstetrics and gynecology interviews and examines Samantha. He learns she ate breakfast before arriving at the hospital. He also learns she has given birth previously while under regional epidural anesthesia without any complications. The resident then reviews the results of electronic fetal monitoring performed after Samantha arrived at the hospital. The EFM tracings continue to be non-reassuring of fetal well-being. No accelerations appear on the EFM, and no fetal movement is otherwise detected.

But the resident mistakenly accepts the labor-and-delivery nurse's chart notation that Samantha came to the hospital for an elective C-section. In addition, he fails to appreciate the urgency of the latest EFM tracings, particularly in light of the results of the non-stress test and truncated biophysical profile performed by her high-risk OB.

Instead, the resident focuses on the fact that Samantha ate breakfast and his belief that she is there on an elective basis. For these reasons, he proposes waiting to perform the C-section – assuming the baby's condition doesn't deteriorate – until six hours after Samantha last ate. He wants to delay delivery to give Samantha time to digest her food before subjecting her to any form of anesthesia. He is particularly concerned that if she is given general anesthesia, it may cause her to vomit into her mask, blocking her airway.

Samantha's panic subsides when she learns her C-section is being postponed for several hours. She assumes her baby must be safe and healthy if the delivery team has decided to wait this long. She assumes wrong. Because she hasn't educated herself about complications that can occur in delivery, she doesn't understand the terminology being used or recognize her baby is at risk. She doesn't know the right questions to ask or the actions to demand. She doesn't even know to insist the hospital's resident consult with her high-risk OB.

Within an hour after Samantha's arrival at the hospital, the resident discusses his proposed delivery plan with the hospital's attending OB, an experienced obstetrician who is in the same obstetrical practice as the high-risk OB who sent Samantha to the hospital for delivery. He must approve the delivery plan before it can be finalized. The attending OB chooses not to come to the patient's bedside to personally assess Samantha's condition and that of her baby. He does not read her medical record or call his partner who sent her for delivery. Without the benefit of any first-hand knowledge of the two patients' conditions, he approves the resident's proposed delivery plan.

Six hours pass since Samantha last ate, but the delivery still is not performed. Approximately a half-hour after the six-hour deadline expires, the hospital staff finally begins to prep her for a C-section. But the six-and-a-half-hour wait proves too stressful for Samantha's baby, whose heart rate plummets to a dangerous level.

An alarm goes out for the attending OB to perform an emergency C-section. He arrives and performs the procedure, but not before Samantha's baby suffers irreversible brain damage as a result of oxygen deprivation. Baby Robert's clinical condition and head imaging studies reveal this sad reality. His brain injury ultimately leads to cerebral palsy and cognitive impairment.

❖   ❖   ❖

It takes more than three years, but suspicions start to creep into Samantha's mind that Robert's brain damage and cerebral palsy could have been avoided. She consults a medical malpractice attorney, who tells her she has no case and politely sends her on her way. But Samantha refuses to give up and finds her way to my firm, Janet, Jenner & Suggs, LLC. We conduct a thorough investigation and identify what we consider gross errors in the obstetrical care Samantha received after arriving at the hospital for delivery.

First, nurses and doctors at the hospital never fully appreciated the true purpose of the admission. They ignored the phone call from the high-risk OB's nurse about why Samantha was being sent to the hospital, as well as the note he sent with her. Inexplicably, they proceeded as if Samantha was admitted for the elective C-section she scheduled before that fateful day when her baby stopped moving. The resident told the attending OB the admission was for an elective procedure when he requested approval to wait up to six hours since the mother's last meal before performing surgery.

It was the attending OB's duty to see Samantha, examine her, and personally review her records. It was his duty to ask the resident probing questions about the patient, and review all the information he had about her and her baby. The attending OB took none of these steps. Essentially, he rubber-stamped the resident's plan. In fact, he didn't see Samantha at any time prior to the call for an emergency C-section.

Had the attending met his obligations, he would have recognized waiting for Samantha's breakfast to digest further was unnecessary and dangerous. He would have known baby Robert urgently needed to be delivered when she was sent to the hospital. The reassessment performed at the hospital did not reveal any signs of improvement. The baby's condition continued to demand urgent delivery. During the six-hour-plus wait that followed admission to the hospital, the baby's condition deteriorated even further. The obstetrical team failed to appreciate that fact, so they waited the full six hours and then some.

No one took into account that the C-section would have been performed under regional, not general, anesthesia. No one took into account that Samantha had previously undergone a C-section using regional anesthesia without any complications arising and without the need to convert to general anesthesia.

Given the lack of fetal movement and the non-reassuring fetal monitor tracings, the risk of severe, irreversible injury to Samantha's baby from delayed delivery far outweighed the comparatively negligible risks associated with any form of anesthesia, despite Samantha's recent food intake.

But these errors were not all we found. The final blow was this: If the doctors had followed their own misguided delivery plan and met their self-imposed six-hour deadline, baby Robert still would have avoided permanent injury. The doctors would have gotten away with their mistakes. Ultimately, it was undisputed that Samantha's baby's irreversible brain damage occurred during the twenty-minute period before his delivery – after the six-hour deadline had expired.

My firm filed suit on behalf of Samantha's child. We could not make a claim on her behalf because the statute of limitations that imposes a time limit on filing such a lawsuit had expired. But we still had ample time to file a lawsuit on behalf of her child. The defendants fought like their lives depended on the outcome of the case, but so did we. We won a record-breaking verdict for baby Robert – one that will provide the compensation he truly deserves and ensure he will be taken care of for the rest of his life.

Lessons from Samantha about Her Rights as a Patient and a Plaintiff

With this experience, Samantha learned important lessons from which all expectant parents would benefit. She learned how to help ensure she and her baby receive the quality medical care they deserve, and she learned their legal rights when that care is lacking.

This young woman will never again place blind faith in an obstetrician or in any physician, for that matter. Her son's birth taught Samantha that relying solely on her doctor for information and advice is not enough; she must take a proactive role in ensuring her next baby is born healthy. She must find ways to expand her obstetrical knowledge base, so she can draw on her own insights, in addition to her doctor's advice, to make a sound decision.

Regrettably, it took a tragedy for Samantha to accept a harsh reality: In the final analysis, she can expect no one – not even her doctor – to share her own level of concern about her health and the health of her baby.

Samantha learned that if she suspects she or her baby may have suffered significant injuries from negligent health care, she should immediately consult an experienced plaintiffs' medical malpractice attorney – one with an established record of success in birth injury litigation. She also learned (to quote Dylan Thomas, though in a different context) to "not go gentle into that good night" if her case is rejected, even by an experienced law firm. She learned that seeking a second legal opinion is every bit as important as seeking a second medical opinion.

The U.S Department of Health & Human Services on Optimizing Health Care Outcomes

The U.S. Department of Health & Human Services strongly agrees patients must be proactive to ensure they receive the quality of health care they deserve. Its Agency for Healthcare Research and Quality alerts all patients to what they can do to help prevent medical errors and stay safe: "The best way to help prevent medical errors is to be an active member of your health care team. That means taking part in every decision about your health care. Research shows that patients who are more involved with their care tend to get better results."

Samantha's conclusions and those of the U.S. Department of Health & Human Services are right on the mark.

21st Century Obstetrical Care

Today, it is more important than ever for expectant parents to obtain medical information from sources other than the treating obstetrician, and be assertive in making decisions about the care the mother and baby receive. This is true, regardless of the parents' socioeconomic status, or the physician's credentials and experience.

The realities of 21st century obstetrical care are far different from those of a generation ago. Too often, obstetricians fall short of the high standards of care your parents enjoyed when they were expecting you. In some respects, the practice of obstetrics has become dysfunctional.

This may seem counterintuitive until you examine the reasons why patient care is suffering. While medical advances have put cutting-edge technologies at the disposal of present-day obstetricians, as is the case with most medical care, the practice of obstetrics has become impersonal and hurried. Doctors are seeing more patients per day and spending less time with each of them.

In today's obstetrical environment, it is not unusual for someone other than the doctor who provided the majority of your prenatal care to deliver your baby. The delivering physician may not be thoroughly familiar with your prenatal history, let alone relevant details of any past pregnancies. In fact, you may never have seen the delivering OB before! This tends to occur in one of two circumstances – a physician from another practice is covering for your off-duty doctor, or a house physician is standing in when your doctor fails to arrive at the hospital in time for delivery.

What other factors account for the current state of obstetrical care?

At the top of the list is a flawed health care system that fails to adequately focus on patient safety. Well more than a decade ago, studies revealed that up to 98,000 patients die, and one million or more patients are injured, each year from medical errors committed in hospitals. As it turns out, these studies appear to have significantly underestimated the number of avoidable deaths. The most recent study estimates the annual death toll to be approximately 400,000. Not enough has been done, or is being done, to improve patient safety.

Another major factor is the flawed system typically used to compensate health care providers, which uses a fee-for-service approach and fails to take into account the quality of the service provided. Those who provide safe care are not rewarded, and those who provide substandard care resulting in patient injuries are not penalized.

In addition, recent economic pressures on the health care system have reduced the number of dollars available to pay health care providers for the services they provide. In many instances, private and government health insurers are paying obstetricians less to deliver babies today than they paid them a decade ago. Doctors get less money, and pregnant women frequently get less care.

To make matters worse, the American Congress of Obstetricians and Gynecologists (ACOG), medical malpractice insurance companies, and hospital risk managers seem to encourage obstetricians to view patients as potential courtroom adversaries. This also contributes to a dysfunctional health care delivery system.

Doctors are among the most respected members of our society, so it may be uncomfortable to question their motives. Moreover, fear of being second-guessed or even sued for malpractice leads some obstetricians to intentionally withhold information from their patients.

If a labor-and-delivery nurse advises your doctor to hurry to the hospital to assess your baby and consider an emergency delivery, and your doctor disagrees, don't expect either of them to tell you about it. Don't expect to be given an opportunity to ask questions and be involved in resolving the disagreement. Don't expect to see an entry in your medical chart about the incident. The Association of Women's

Health, Obstetrical and Neonatal Nurses (AWHONN) acknowledges the regrettable reality that obstetrical nurses are privately discouraged from "advertising" conflicts of this nature.

Yet another factor – although not unique to the 21st century – is that many physicians tend to believe their patients are incapable of understanding complex medical issues. This may be pure condescension, or it may reflect a reluctance to dedicate the time required to explain health care issues thoroughly. Either way, it is unacceptable. In matters affecting your health and that of your baby, you have a right to expect full disclosure.

Choosing Reliable Sources of Information

Like Samantha, many expectant mothers today realize they cannot count on their obstetricians to inform them fully about their routine care, let alone how to avoid or limit the effects of potentially life-threatening complications. In record numbers, expectant mothers and fathers are turning to other sources of information to become better educated about obstetrical care. The most common among them include birthing classes, the Internet, and books about pregnancy and delivery.

But do these other sources adequately pick up the slack? After all, finding supplemental educational information you can trust is as crucial as recognizing the need for it in the first place.

Lamaze®-type birthing classes use an almost mystical approach to birthing education. They encourage pregnant women to trust their "inner wisdom" to guide them through birth. Make no mistake – Lamaze® and similar birthing classes serve an important function. They help expectant parents understand the birthing process, teach valuable techniques for easing the pain of labor and delivery, and help fathers or partners take an active role in pregnancy and childbirth. Birthing classes can be memorable and empowering. Educating parents-to-be about potentially serious obstetrical complications, however, is not the focus of their curriculum.

Without discounting the importance of a mother's intuition, you need to be able to call on something more substantial than instinct in a case of obstetrical emergency. That's when alternative education becomes critical.

Turning to the Internet for reliable obstetrical information presents its own challenges and pitfalls. First, much of the information online originates from complex obstetrical textbooks and journals written for doctors, not patients. Second, even the material that is coherent is sometimes contradictory. Most importantly, just as with newspapers, you cannot always believe what you read on the Internet. Some medical literature is unreliable – even articles that appear on seemingly credible websites.

Now, take off your rose-colored glasses for a moment and think about it: in birth injury lawsuits, the stakes are extremely high. Juries typically decide whether to award babies and their parents the millions of dollars needed to provide a lifetime of care. Much of the evidence juries consider in arriving at their verdicts draws on obstetrical literature. Knowing this, some obstetricians have written articles that give false impressions about the quality of care 21st century obstetricians deliver to their patients. Lawyers who defend obstetricians sued for malpractice lean heavily on this tainted literature in their efforts to sway jurors in favor of defendants and their malpractice carriers. Avoiding accountability for negligence is the objective.

Case in point: many lawsuits turn on whether the obstetrician accurately interpreted electronic fetal heart monitoring results. Like the EKG used to detect heart dysfunction in adults, EFM monitors the baby's heart rate patterns. The patterns are displayed on a monitor and appear on paper tracings. Through variations in its heart rate, the baby communicates to the world outside the womb, particularly the obstetrical staff, about a vital aspect of his or her health – most notably, whether there is reason for concern about the amount of oxygen being pumped to the baby's brain. In essence, EFM enables a fetus to "speak from the heart" to sound an alarm.

As a means of combating these cases, some obstetricians have authored literature that unjustifiably implies EFM tracings are frequently not worth the paper they are printed on. Some articles even suggest tracings are so difficult to interpret, obstetricians should not be held responsible for misreading them unless the results are extremely and obviously abnormal. Routinely, defense lawyers rely on these purposely slanted articles to try to convince jurors to side with their clients.

Fortunately for victims of obstetrical negligence, some of the world's most renowned obstetricians are not prejudiced against birth injury plaintiffs. These doctors have set the record straight about EFM in courtrooms across the country, backing up their testimony with experience and credible studies. They consistently maintain that tracings do not need to flatline or plunge to dangerously low levels with every contraction before obstetricians should recognize the baby is seriously at risk from lack of oxygen. They scoff at the absurdity that obstetricians are only trained to appreciate and respond to blatantly obvious irregularities.

Books about pregnancy and delivery are another popular alternative source of information for expectant parents. One of the most well-known books is *What to Expect® When You're Expecting*, which has sold millions of copies. Although the book contains a great deal of helpful information, it doesn't give the attention to potential obstetrical complications a pregnant woman needs and deserves. Further, it omits critical information about when and how to be proactive.

It appears the authors of *What to Expect® When You're Expecting* foolishly tried to fill the gaps in their own obstetrical knowledge by relying heavily on ACOG literature. This organization doesn't advocate for patients; it advocates for doctors! The organization spends huge sums of money each year lobbying politicians to support legislation intended to drastically limit the rights of victims of substandard obstetrical care – victims just like Samantha and her baby.

The American Congress of Obstetricians and Gynecologists' bias in favor of doctors appears to have infected the authors of *What To Expect® When You're Expecting*. The book devotes only a single chapter to obstetrical complications, as if they are not important, and the authors preface the chapter with this statement: "If you've had a problem-free pregnancy so far, though, this need-to-know chapter is not for you (you don't need to know any of it)...Skip it and save yourself some unneeded worry."

The book your doctor wants you to read encourages you to put your head in the sand and ignore even the possibility of life-threatening complications! Keeping you in the dark is wrong. Educating you about problems before they occur is your best defense against serious injury to you and your baby.

We're on Your Side

Patients' Rights and Doctors' Wrongs® – Secrets to a Safer Pregnancy and Childbirth provides essential, trustworthy, easily understandable educational information and advice that has not been readily available to expectant parents until now. And it presents this material from the perspective of protecting the well-being of babies and their parents, not doctors – an approach that has been lacking in medical literature, birthing classes, on the Internet, or in any other format available to expectant parents.

This book talks about the uncomfortable reality that serious problems sometimes develop during pregnancy. It arms you with the information you need to be prepared for those complications and react to them based on a foundation of knowledge, thereby minimizing their consequences. We present this information in the context of real-life incidents. However, the names of parents and children have been changed.

Patients' Rights and Doctors' Wrongs® – Secrets to a Safer Pregnancy and Childbirth equips you to be an informed consumer of obstetrical care. In reality, the more informed you are, the more you will be able to protect your baby and help your obstetrician give you better care. The authors are two professionals who have extensive expertise in evaluating the quality of obstetrical care.

Giles H. Manley is a board certified obstetrician-gynecologist with twenty years of experience in obstetrics. Dr. Manley has delivered more than 2,000 babies, and he has served as an expert witness on behalf of both plaintiffs and defendants in obstetrical malpractice lawsuits. Dr. Manley is now an attorney, and works hand-in-hand with Howard A. Janet, advocating for victims of obstetrical and other medical negligence. Super Lawyers®, a renowned attorney peer review organization, recognizes Dr. Manley as a "Rising Star" in the field of medical malpractice law.

Howard A. Janet is widely recognized as one of the nation's foremost plaintiffs' birth injury attorneys. Over the course of his more than thirty years in the field of medical malpractice, he has been consulted about more than 20,000 instances of possible obstetrical malpractice. On numerous occasions, his insight in the field of obstetrical negligence has helped him uncover errors missed by other highly regarded lawyers. But Mr. Janet doesn't stop with identifying meritorious cases; in the courtroom and at the settlement table, he has achieved record-breaking results that provide families with the peace of mind they need and deserve. One of the country's most respected attorney peer-review organizations, *The Best Lawyers in America*®, honored Mr. Janet as a "Lawyer of the Year" in 2012 and 2015. Another leading peer-review organization, Martindale-Hubble®, has consistently awarded him the highest rating possible (AV) for professional competence and ethics.

More comprehensive biographical information about the authors can be found in Part XII, entitled "About the Authors."

Together, Dr. Manley and Mr. Janet give you a comprehensive, candid perspective on pregnancy and childbirth. The information contained in these pages has the potential to help avoid devastating, life-altering injuries and save countless lives.

Here is their message to you, mothers- and fathers-to-be:

If you want obstetrical information that will help you obtain the high-quality care you deserve, then you have found it. If you want sound guidance that will help you navigate the sea of false, deceptive, contradictory material that is out there, this is it. If you want to be treated as a responsible, intelligent adult – instead of being patted on the head and told, "Don't worry, be happy" – you have come to the right place.

We readily admit it: we are on your side. We are biased in favor of patients and patients' rights. In this book, we don't pull any punches. We don't hold back at the risk of offending the obstetrical establishment. Our goal is simple: healthy mothers and healthy babies. We are shining a spotlight on potential complications – not to cause you undue worry, but to help you understand why it is so important to be fully informed about your obstetrical care.

In malpractice litigation, obstetricians can avoid liability if they have met the minimum standards expected of a reasonably prudent physician. That is the law. But we believe expectant mothers and their babies are entitled to more. If that means raising the bar for doctors, so be it.

Complications arise during pregnancy and childbirth in a variety of circumstances. Samantha's story is just one example. The list of complications that can occur is long, with abruptions, uterine ruptures, infections, and maternal hypertension among the most serious. *Patients' Rights and Doctors' Wrongs® – Secrets to a Safer Pregnancy and Childbirth* addresses these and many other problems that can have potentially dire consequences for you and your baby.

Permanent injuries from dangerous complications can include neurologic injuries of the type Samantha's son sustained, lesser brain injuries that cause learning disabilities, or nerve injuries that impair the functions of a baby's arm or shoulder. Thankfully, they can often be avoided through appropriate, timely intervention. Recognizing the warning signs and taking the proper action immediately can turn a potentially devastating complication into a mere speed bump on the highway to a safe delivery.

Most likely, both you and your baby will come through pregnancy and childbirth just fine even in the 21st century. But we urge you not to take a problem-free experience for granted. Remember and heed the old adage, "An ounce of prevention is worth a pound of cure."

PART II

Waking Up to Possible Side Effects of Epidurals and Other Types of Regional Anesthesia

CHAPTER 1

Michelle's Story

As she is wheeled into the operating room (OR), Michelle braces to the rush of cold air and squints into the harsh glare of the overhead lights. She is familiar with the delivery room. This is her second baby and her second C-section. As the orderlies position and drape her, she glances around at the equipment and staff. The entire obstetrical team is busily preparing for what they expect to be an uncomplicated delivery. Her heart races with excitement.

It is 7:30 p.m. Michelle has been at the hospital since a little after midnight, when she was admitted because of ongoing contractions. She wasn't officially in labor, and she won't be until her cervix either begins to dilate or efface.

Michelle is thirty-eight weeks pregnant, far enough along to be considered full-term. Her obstetrician has scheduled a C-section at thirty-eight and one-half weeks, with delivery to be moved up only if Michelle's contractions produce cervical changes. Meanwhile, the plan is to monitor her baby's well-being and observe Michelle for signs of labor.

The initial electronic fetal monitoring tracings showed her baby was doing fine. Throughout the day, little Tanya's heartbeat has remained strong. The labor and delivery staff continued the fetal monitoring until just after 6:00 p.m., about the time Michelle's obstetrician arrived at the hospital.

Now, after about twenty hours of contractions, Michelle's cervix has dilated, indicating she is in labor. Three more hours go by without significant change. Her OB diagnoses an arrest of labor and calls for a C-section. Her baby will be born tonight! Bone-tired and in pain, she focuses on her breathing and the thought that the worst of her labor is likely over.

Behind Michelle, the anesthesiologist prepares to administer the epidural in preparation for the C-section. Michelle breathes deeply. *I've done this before. I know what to expect. In a few minutes the pain will be gone, and my daughter will be in my arms.*

At 7:40 p.m., the anesthesiologist administers the epidural injection. Michelle feels pressure as the needle slips between her vertebrae. Almost instantly, she senses the familiar prickling sensation in her toes. A moment later, her abdomen and pelvic area begin to tingle. As the pain eases, she begins to relax.

But Michelle's serenity is fleeting. Shortly after receiving the injection, a sickening wave of nausea washes over her. Her stomach turns, and her throat fills with bile. Everything and everyone around her begins to spin.

Michelle knows this feeling. It is the same nausea and lightheadedness she experienced when her blood pressure dropped sharply just after she received an epidural for the delivery of her first baby. Her obstetrician and anesthesiologist are aware it happened before, and should be watching for it with this delivery.

Michelle searches the faces in the room for her obstetrician, but he is not there. The only doctor she sees is the anesthesiologist, who confirms her low blood pressure and gives her medication that elevates it within ten to fifteen minutes. "Don't worry," he says. "We're monitoring you closely. We've got it under control."

Minutes crawl by like hours. Finally, Michelle's obstetrician enters the OR and bends over his patient. "Are you ready, Michelle? Let's deliver your baby girl."

Baby Tanya is born at 8:34 p.m. From the moment of birth, it is obvious her appearance and behavior are not normal. She is not crying or moving, and she is terribly pale. Tanya's heart rate, respiration, muscle tone, skin color, and response to stimuli are all extremely deficient.

Within the first twenty-four hours of life, Tanya develops seizures – a telltale sign she has suffered a brain injury from lack of oxygen shortly before delivery. Over the first year of life, Tanya exhibits concerning signs of developmental delay. It isn't long before she is formally diagnosed with cerebral palsy.

CHAPTER 2

What Went Wrong and Why

Introduction

Michelle's story sheds light on the most common complications that occur when expectant mothers receive regional anesthesia – maternal hypotension (abnormally low blood pressure) and slowing of the fetal heart rate. Mothers experience hypotension in 25 to 40 percent of pregnancies. Babies develop non-reassuring fetal heart rate patterns up to 25 percent of the time, necessitating approximately 2,000 emergency C-sections each year in the United States. When obstetrical and anesthesia personnel exercise the requisite degree of vigilance, permanent injury to baby and mother can be avoided.

This chapter and the one that follows explain what constitutes the proper degree of vigilance. They also point out the kinds of avoidable mistakes to which some mothers and babies can be subjected. The information that follows will empower you to ensure your health care providers take the necessary measures to protect your baby's well-being and your own.

Unrecognized Complication

Two serious complications developed soon after Michelle received epidural anesthesia for her C-section, but the medical providers in the OR recognized and corrected only one – Michelle's sharp decline in blood pressure. The other complication, a dangerous drop in baby Tanya's heart rate, went unnoticed and uncorrected until after her birth.

The OR staff did nothing about it because they didn't *know* about it. They didn't know because they didn't check. In fact, no one monitored the baby's heart rate for the entire period Michelle was in the operating room – not before the epidural, not after the injection, and not even after her hypotensive episode.

Despite an order given by the obstetrician for continuous electronic fetal heart monitoring, the obstetrical nurses discontinued EFM a full hour and a half before Michelle was moved to the operating room. They never resumed it. Michelle's obstetrician wasn't even present in the operating room when her epidural was administered.

Both maternal hypotension and a dangerously low drop in the baby's heart rate are undesirable side-effects that can occur following the administration of epidural anesthesia for a C-section. The chance of the baby's heart rate falling to an unsafe level exists even if the mother does not become hypotensive. That risk increases when the mother experiences a hypotensive episode. But in Michelle's case, even the mother's hypotensive episode failed to trigger an assessment of baby Tanya's heart rate.

Once the mother's blood pressure returns to a normal level, the potential for crisis is not over. There is no guarantee the baby's heart rate will return to normal, even if the mother's blood pressure normalizes. To be certain of the baby's well-being following administration of epidural anesthesia for a C-section, regardless of whether the mother becomes hypotensive, either external fetal monitoring or internal monitoring should be continued virtually up until the moment of birth.

If external fetal monitoring is being used, it should be continued until the mother's abdomen has been sterilized with antiseptic solution, and delivery should be completed within several minutes thereafter. With internal monitoring – which does not pose the same concerns about contaminating the sterile surgical field as external fetal monitoring – there is no reason to discontinue monitoring until the OB begins the C-section.

While Tanya's heart pumped at a dangerously slow pace, her brain and other vital organs were being deprived of an adequate flow of oxygen. Because of the extensive amount of time that elapsed from the onset of this complication until the time of delivery, Tanya sustained permanently life-altering brain damage. The C-section should have been started, at the very latest, when her mother's blood pressure normalized. The procedure would have been completed within several minutes, and Tanya would have escaped any permanent impairment.

Inexcusable Oversights

Inexcusable oversights by Michelle's obstetrical and anesthesia teams, poor communication between the two teams, and faulty hospital policy – all were responsible for the tragic turn of events shortly before Tanya's birth that changed her life forever.

The actions and inactions of Michelle's delivery team and the hospital were completely contrary to even the most minimal standards expected today.

The Obstetrical Team

The obstetrician bears responsibility for failing to be in the delivery room when the anesthesiologist gave the epidural injection. He checked on Michelle and her baby when he arrived at the hospital just after 6:00 p.m., but never looked in on them again until he was called to perform the C-section. If he had, he would have realized the baby's status was unknown – an extremely unsafe circumstance. Further, although he knew an epidural takes effect within approximately ten to fifteen minutes, he never investigated why more than double that amount of time passed before he was called to surgery.

Michelle's obstetrician also failed to ensure both Michelle's and Tanya's reactions to the epidural would be monitored.

Finally, when he did arrive in the delivery room, the obstetrician neglected to ask about the condition of either mother or baby. He assumed both of them were being monitored closely and he would be told if there were any complications. In view of his knowledge about the hospital's policies and practices with respect to staffing the OR for C-sections, he lacked any reasonable basis to make such an assumption.

Hospital Policies and Procedures

Those very staffing policies and practices, which fell well below generally accepted hospital standards, substantially factored into the failure to adequately monitor Tanya's state of health in the OR. As a matter of policy and practice, the hospital did not require monitoring fetal well-being following administration of an epidural for C-section. Once Michelle was in the operating room, there was no way to monitor her baby's well-being, as the hospital failed to equip the OR with an EFM or a Doppler/Doptone (a hand-held ultrasound device that gives a digital readout of the FHR).

Consistent with the hospital's substandard policies and procedures, the nurse in the operating room was concerned only with preparing Michelle for surgery. She was not charged with the responsibility of performing fetal monitoring, and the hospital provided her no means by which to accomplish it. Tanya was unmonitored the entire time she was in the delivery room. And that followed on the heels of the obstetrical nurse's failure to monitor her for the previous ninety minutes.

The Anesthesia Team

The members of the anesthesia team completely disregarded their second patient, baby Tanya. They recognized Michelle's hypotensive episode and took appropriate steps to correct it, but they failed to address the potentially dangerous effects it could have on her baby. They turned a blind eye to the baby's well-being, even though they knew there was no fetal monitoring equipment in the OR.

Michelle's anesthesiologist and the nurse anesthetist assisting him knew about the hospital's deficient monitoring policy and observed that no one in the delivery room was monitoring Tanya. They knew the baby could develop adverse side effects from the epidural her mother received. Nevertheless, they accepted those circumstances and subjected Tanya to the associated risk.

Their conduct became even more indefensible once they became aware of Michelle's hypotension – a clear signal the dangers to Tanya had increased. They did not coordinate fetal monitoring, and they did not immediately summon Michelle's obstetrician, who was within ear-shot of the delivery room. After Michelle's obstetrician finally arrived in the OR, neither the anesthesiologist nor the nurse anesthetist informed him about the drop in Michelle's blood pressure. Oblivious to Tanya's condition and the hypotensive episode Michelle had experienced, the obstetrician proceeded with the C-section in a routine manner instead of delivering her emergently, as the circumstances required.

Failure to Inform

Michelle knew the signs and symptoms of hypotension from her previous delivery, but she had no knowledge of its potential effects on her unborn child. Her first baby had been able to tolerate the regional anesthesia and his mother's hypotension. If Michelle had been adequately informed of the risk regional anesthesia for C-section poses to babies, she would have insisted her baby be adequately monitored and delivered without undue delay. She would have known it wasn't enough for the OR staff to monitor and care solely for her.

CHAPTER 3

What Expectant Mothers Should Know

The Basics

Regional anesthesia eliminates the expectant mother's sensation of pain in the abdomen, pelvis and genital area, and also affects the legs. The three classes of regional anesthetics include local anesthetics (usually bupivicaine or lidocaine); narcotics (such as morphine); or a combination of both. Forms of regional anesthesia include epidural, spinal and spinal-epidural. In the case of an epidural, a hypodermic needle is inserted between two vertebrae into the fatty space surrounding the spinal cord. With a spinal, the needle is inserted into the fluid-filled sac just beyond the fatty space.

The mother remains fully awake during the injection. She either assumes a fetal-like position, or leans forward from a seated posture on the bed or operating room table. These positions are necessary to open the space between the lumbar vertebrae, allowing safe placement of the needle. The anesthetic is injected into either the fatty space or spinal fluid, where nerves controlling sensation in the lower abdomen, pelvis and legs emerge. In the case of a spinal-epidural, the anesthetic is injected at both sites.

All regional anesthetics numb the nerves at the injection site. However, the anesthetic also tends to travel both upward and downward from the point of injection, suppressing sensation not only in the pelvic area, but also in the upper abdomen and legs. This traveling can be controlled somewhat by the amount of drug used and the mother's physical positioning. The anesthesiologist should assess how far the anesthetic has traveled by testing different areas of the mother's abdomen and chest to ensure the level is safe and correct.

Often, the anesthetic affects not only the sensory nerves, giving pain relief, but also the motor nerves. This makes it impossible for the mother to move her legs. As the anesthetic's effects move upward, the mother may experience the sensation of breathing difficulty. This feeling can be frightening, but it is entirely normal. Prior to the injection, the anesthesiologist should place a device called a *pulse oximeter* on the mother's finger to measure the oxygen level in her blood and ensure she is in no danger.

If you encounter difficulty breathing following the administration of anesthesia, remember: as long as you are talking, you are breathing appropriately.

Epidural for C-Section or Labor

During both C-section and labor, an epidural can relieve pain and desensitize the abdomen and pelvis. Its onset is fairly slow, taking up to fifteen minutes to give complete relief. This form of regional anesthesia can be administered in either of two ways. When given as a single large dose, the epidural provides relief for a period of thirty minutes to twenty-four hours, depending on the type of anesthetic used. When given continuously through a catheter, it gives pain relief until delivery, whether that takes place in one hour or in forty-eight hours.

Up to 90 percent of mothers receive an epidural during labor. It is also frequently used during C-sections. The volume of the drug injected into the fatty space surrounding the spinal cord controls its distribution. Even so, the anesthetic occasionally does not spread to all the desired areas, resulting in incomplete or uneven pain relief.

Spinal for C-Section

The spinal injection is used almost exclusively during C-sections. It has a very fast onset, usually providing pain relief within minutes. This form of regional anesthesia is administered as a single dose injected into the fluid that surrounds the spinal cord. It works the same way as the epidural, by numbing the nerves surrounding the injection site.

Because it is injected into a fluid-filled space, the distribution of the spinal anesthetic is virtually always complete. As with an epidural, the duration of relief depends on the type of anesthetic used. Often, a combination of narcotic and local anesthesia is used. The local anesthetic eliminates both pain and motor function, but it is short-acting. The narcotic affects only sensory function and lasts as long as twenty-four hours. This allows the mother mobility shortly after her C-section and provides pain relief without drowsiness for the first day.

Spinal-Epidural for C-Section

A spinal-epidural is a combination of the two types of regional anesthesia just described. Also administered by injection between the vertebrae, the spinal-epidural is accomplished with only a single needle stick. It is a little more difficult to perform, but has the benefits of a rapid onset and long, controlled duration.

Operating Room Versus Labor Room

The steps involved in administering regional anesthesia to a laboring mother are almost identical to those outlined above for a mother undergoing a C-section. However, there is one major difference – the area of the hospital where the regional anesthesia is administered.

When receiving regional anesthesia in the operating room, if an emergency arises, the patient is already on the operating room table, the surgical instruments are ready for use, and converting to general anesthesia can be accomplished without delay. On the other hand, when the epidural is administered during labor, the patient is usually several minutes away from the operating room, and the obstetrician and OR staff may not be readily available. The delays caused by these circumstances can cost precious minutes during which the baby's brain needs oxygen.

Should an emergency arise, the health care team should be capable of performing a C-section within ten to fifteen minutes after the onset of the emergency – not within a half-hour, as suggested in published obstetrical literature.

Risks Associated With Regional Anesthesia

Risks to Mother

Maternal hypotension is by far the most common side-effect of all forms of regional anesthesia. This condition is defined as a significant drop in the mother's blood pressure – a 25 percent drop from her baseline level or a 30 percent drop from the pre-anesthesia level. The baseline level is the average blood pressure for several hours prior to injection. The pre-anesthesia level just prior to injection tends to be a little higher, as the mother is nervous and in pain.

However, any drop in the mother's blood pressure can be significant because not all patients react to regional anesthesia the same way. Both the extent of the decrease and the mother's reaction to it depend on her intravascular volume – the amount of fluid flowing through her blood vessels to her heart. The greater the volume, the less likely hypotension will occur. That is why a patient should be given at least a liter of IV fluids prior to administering regional anesthesia.

Hypotensive episodes are experienced by about 25 to 40 percent of regional anesthesia patients. This side-effect can develop within minutes of the injection or up to an hour later. The most common sign of maternal hypotension is the sudden onset of nausea and/or vomiting.

Another possible side-effect the mother may experience with any form of regional anesthesia is the spinal headache. The fluid surrounding the spinal cord and brain is contained within a single sac that runs the length of the spinal cord. Occasionally, the epidural needle advances too far and pierces this sac, allowing spinal fluid to leak from it and depleting the amount of fluid around the brain. This produces a severe headache in the mother, especially when she is in an upright position. Spinal headaches occur less frequently with spinal anesthesia because the needle used for a spinal is much smaller than the one used for an epidural. This smaller needle causes such a small puncture that the sac surrounding the spinal fluid normally closes over it.

Potential side-effects of puncturing the spinal sac include direct nerve damage (the needle hits and damages one of the nerves), paralysis, and infection. These are extremely rare and should not deter a mother from undergoing regional anesthesia.

Risks to Baby

When the mother's blood pressure drops, her body shifts the flow of oxygen-laden blood away from the uterus and toward her own vital organs, taking oxygen away from the placenta and the fetus. About 10 percent of the time, this causes the baby's heart rate to drop below one hundred beats per minute. (The normal range is 110 to 160 beats per minute.) When this condition lasts for ten minutes or more, it is called *bradycardia*. Rarely, a significant drop in the baby's heart rate can occur as a direct result of the anesthetic alone. In the overwhelming majority of cases, significant slowing of the baby's heart rate is only temporary. The fetal heart rate usually returns to normal, with no ill effects on the baby. However, if the condition persists for a prolonged period of time, the consequences can be devastating.

A healthy baby can often tolerate a near-total decrease in oxygen for about ten to fifteen minutes without beginning to suffer permanent brain injury. The longer the baby is deprived of an adequate flow of oxygen, the more serious the consequences.

If a prolonged bradycardia occurs in your baby, immediate delivery is crucial to avoid brain injury. Once delivered, the baby relies on breathing, not the mother's blood, for the oxygen its brain and other organs need. Breathing can be assisted once the baby is delivered, if necessary. Also, after delivery, various direct measures are available to restore the baby's heart rate to an acceptable level.

When Complications Arise

Corrective Measures for Mother

The severity of the hypotensive episode dictates the action anesthesia personnel should take to restore the mother's blood pressure to an acceptable level. This may merely involve intensifying steps used to prevent maternal hypotension from developing in the first place.

As a purely precautionary measure before any maternal hypotension is detected, the anesthesiologist usually has the mother lean slightly toward her left side. This takes pressure off the aorta and vena cava, which carry oxygenated blood from the heart to all the body's organs and limbs, and return it to be re-oxygenated. These *great vessels* are located slightly to the right of the spinal column. The weight of the uterus and the fetus it contains can compress the great vessels, limiting the volume of blood that circulates through them. Leaning the mother to the left relieves this compression and restores full blood flow. When a drop in the mother's blood pressure is detected, the first step is to exaggerate the left-sided tilt in the mother's position.

The second appropriate step to relieve maternal hypotension is to increase the rate and amount of IV fluids she is receiving. This raises the volume of blood flowing through the blood vessels and helps return the mother's blood pressure to normal. It is another example of taking the precautionary administration of IV fluids to a higher level. In many cases, these are the only steps necessary to correct maternal hypotension and prevent harm to the baby.

When changing position and increasing IV fluids fail to normalize the mother's blood pressure, the anesthesiologist or nurse anesthetist will turn to medication. Typically, ephedrine is administered through the mother's IV. This medication causes the smooth muscles surrounding the blood vessels to contract, increasing blood pressure. Ephedrine usually takes effect fairly rapidly, within less than a minute. Several additional doses may be necessary to fully restore the mother's blood pressure.

Corrective Measures for Baby

Fortunately, relieving hypotension in the mother almost always corrects bradycardia in the baby. But never forget the significance of the word *almost*. Further, do not lose sight of the possibility the regional anesthetic may cause the fetal heart rate to decrease to a dangerous level.

Administering oxygen to the mother via face mask is another protective step that can be taken to prevent complications related to regional anesthesia. This increases the amount of oxygen in the mother's blood, as well as oxygen flow to the baby.

Before taking corrective measures, as opposed to preventive measures, the obstetrical staff should confirm the baby's heart rate has actually dropped. Often, they place a scalp electrode on the baby's head (called *internal electronic fetal monitoring*) to obtain a more accurate heart rate reading than is possible with an external monitor. If this step cannot be accomplished or the accuracy of the scalp electrode is in question, a portable ultrasound unit can be used to view a real-time image of the baby's heart.

If an unsafe drop in the baby's heart rate is confirmed following regional anesthesia, regardless of whether the mother has experienced a hypotensive episode, the OB team should intensify precautionary measures (just as when attempting to correct the mother's hypotension). Appropriate corrective steps include repositioning the mother, increasing her fluids, administering an additional large amount of fluid a "bolus," and further increasing her oxygen. No more than several minutes should be devoted to these corrective measures. If these measures fail to return the baby's heart rate to an acceptable level within just a few minutes, a true emergency is unfolding, and the baby must be delivered immediately.

When It's Time to Deliver, Time Is of the Essence

Responding quickly to bradycardia is essential because even a well-oxygenated baby can tolerate this condition for only about ten to fifteen minutes before suffering permanent brain damage. If the fetal heart rate drops significantly after the injection of a regional anesthetic for C-section and efforts fail to resuscitate the baby immediately, an emergency delivery must be performed.

If the regional anesthesia has not taken full effect or is not expected to take effect imminently, a general anesthetic should be administered to avoid delaying delivery. Regardless of the form of anesthesia used, once it is evident the baby is at serious risk and the mother is adequately anesthetized, the baby should be delivered within approximately five minutes. In an emergency, ordinarily, no more than about two to three minutes should elapse between the time of the skin incision and the uterine incision, and no more than about one to three minutes should elapse between the time of the uterine incision and delivery. Often, delivery can be accomplished within one to two minutes after the start of the operation.

Whenever a C-section is being performed, a swift delivery is important. After the surgeon cuts into the uterus, the mother's blood (which is the baby's source of oxygen) is no longer flowing to the baby.

Absent adequate oxygen, acid builds up in the baby's blood, a condition known as *acidosis*. If acidosis is allowed to persist for an extended period of time, the baby's brain tissue is at risk of being permanently damaged. Time is truly of the essence.

In some rare instances, a significant accumulation of scar tissue from prior surgeries can cause surgery to take more than the desired five-minute time period. If the baby is in good condition with no ill effects from anesthesia or some other complicating factor, a safe delivery is still likely. However, if no adhesions are present, there is no credible excuse for delay.

When a persistent, significant drop in the baby's heart rate develops in response to an epidural given for pain relief during labor, the mother should be moved to the operating room without delay. If the baby's heart rate recovers, the mother should be monitored in the operating room for about thirty minutes. Assuming the baby's heart rate continues to be reassuring during that time period, the mother can be returned to her labor room. On the other hand, if the baby's heart rate remains dangerously low, an emergency delivery should be performed.

Always determine the experience level of the surgeon performing your C-section. The higher the potential for a complicated delivery, the more experience your surgeon needs.

Monitoring Two Patients, Not One

There are two patients in the labor and delivery suite – mother and baby – and the importance of monitoring them both cannot be overstressed. Ideally, this dual monitoring should be maintained throughout labor and delivery, but if this is not possible, monitoring the baby should resume immediately after birth. The stress of labor can quicken the effects of regional anesthesia on the baby, but anesthesia alone can be equally dangerous to the baby of a non-laboring mother undergoing a scheduled C-section.

Monitoring the Mother

Once the mother is on the operating table, several monitoring devices are used to keep tabs on her status and ensure her safety. A blood pressure cuff is placed around her upper arm and connected to an electronic monitor, with the digital read-out easily visible to all members of the health care team. The cuff automatically inflates every few minutes prior to administration of the regional anesthetic, and every one to two minutes after the anesthetic is injected. This process continues until the start of surgery.

Not all mothers experience the same physical responses to anesthesia. To ensure the mother is sufficiently numb for surgery, the anesthesiology team uses tactile stimulation (gauging response to the sense of touch) and verbal communication. The anesthesiologist tests various parts of the mother's abdomen and pelvic area by touching them with a pinprick or alcohol swab. He also questions her carefully about whether and where she may be experiencing tingling sensations, as well as whether she feels nauseous or lightheaded – symptoms of the onset of hypotension.

Once surgery is underway, as long as no complications arise, such as profuse bleeding, the anesthesia staff continues monitoring the mother's blood pressure at slightly longer intervals (about every five minutes) until she is transferred to the recovery room.

In recovery, the mother's blood pressure is monitored every ten to fifteen minutes. Just as before injection of the epidural, a pulse oximeter is placed on one of the mother's fingers to measure the oxygenation of her blood and her heart rate, or pulse. Both the blood pressure monitoring and the pulse oximeter remain in place until the mother leaves recovery and is taken to the postpartum floor. If additional oxygen is needed, it is administered either by facemask or nasal cannula (two small plastic prongs placed in the nostrils).

Monitoring the Baby

Clearly, the safety of the unborn child is equally as important as that of the mother. The baby's well-being can be safeguarded most easily by starting surgery within five to seven minutes after the injection of the regional anesthetic. In any event, the safest course is to monitor the baby's heart rate patterns as long as possible until delivery. This gives insight into the adequacy of the baby's oxygen level and the extent to which the baby is at risk of harm by remaining in the uterus.

Electronic monitoring of the fetal heart can be done either continuously, with an internal or external EFM device, or intermittently, with a Doptone (a hand-held ultrasound device that gives a digital readout). Internal EFM is accomplished by attaching an electrode to the baby's head, which is possible only after the rupture of the mother's bag of water. External EFM is performed by attaching an electrode to the mother's abdomen. (These procedures are detailed in the chapter devoted to electronic fetal monitoring.)

In high-risk pregnancies, continuous EFM is required. In other pregnancies, prevailing standards of care permit intermittent fetal assessment with a Doptone for thirty seconds at five- to ten- minute intervals. We urge you to insist on the preferred method, continuous EFM, which provides an ongoing, uninterrupted stream of information about the baby's condition.

Whichever method is used, at minimum, it should be continued until the anesthetic reaches a level allowing the start of surgery. This ensures detection of any bradycardic episode lasting more than about two minutes. If electronic fetal heart monitoring reveals prolonged bradycardia, it takes only a few minutes to induce general anesthesia – more than enough time to deliver the baby safely.

Once sterile prep of the mother's abdomen has begun, it is no longer possible to continue monitoring the baby unless internal EFM is in place. For this reason, the abdomen should not be prepped until the anesthesiologist signals the correct level of anesthesia for surgery has been reached.

The same care and precautions taken to monitor and protect the baby in the labor suite should be taken in the operating room.

Responsibilities of Your Health Care Team

The Obstetrical Team

At minimum, the obstetrical team should include a surgeon, a surgical assistant, and a circulating nurse trained in fetal heart rate monitoring. Ideally, two obstetrical nurses should be present. The team should also include a scrub technician responsible for handing the surgical instruments to the doctor.

Before the start of surgery, a nurse and technician count the surgical instruments and sponges. If there is only one circulating nurse, this count should be completed prior to the induction of anesthesia, freeing the nurse to perform fetal monitoring during the critical period after anesthesia is administered. At the conclusion of surgery, the surgical instruments and sponges are counted again to ensure nothing was left in the patient's abdomen.

The circulating nurse is also responsible for preparing the patient for surgery, summoning the pediatric team to the OR, ensuring the instrument used to cauterize tissue is operating properly, and grounding the patient to prevent burns.

The obstetrician performing the surgery should be in the room to assist with monitoring, calming the patient, and ensuring she is positioned correctly. Once it is clear the anesthesia has been administered correctly and is working properly, the obstetrician should begin the surgery. The obstetrical assistant should already be in the OR – gowned, gloved, and ready to assist with surgery.

Let us emphasize once more: the administration of anesthesia is a potentially high-risk procedure. The entire obstetrical team must be present in the operating room when it is being performed.

The Anesthesia Team

The anesthesia team consists of an anesthesiologist, a nurse anesthetist, or both. They are responsible for the safe administration of regional anesthesia. This includes proper placement and dosing of the regional anesthetic, providing oxygen and hydration for the mother, and monitoring her vital signs.

The primary responsibility of the anesthesia team is to monitor the mother for signs of hypotension. They should monitor her blood pressure every minute, from the time regional anesthesia is given until the start of surgery. Should she become hypotensive, the anesthesia team must correct her condition with IV fluids and/or medication, and notify the obstetrical team.

The anesthesia team's second major concern is achieving and maintaining the correct level of anesthesia. They confirm this in a variety of ways, the most important of which is by communicating with the patient. By using tactile stimulation and questioning the mother closely about the sensations she is feeling, they can get a very good idea of the level of anesthesia. If necessary, they can adjust the level by changing the position of the bed or, if an epidural is used, administering more medication. If it becomes necessary to switch to general anesthesia, the anesthesia team is also responsible for accomplishing that process safely.

The Importance of Communication

The key to practicing safe medicine is good communication among health care providers. Complications rarely result in serious injuries when communication is optimum.

Again, the two major concerns with regional anesthesia for a C-section are hypotension in the mother and bradycardia in the baby. Anytime the mother's blood pressure drops to a level requiring administration of fluids or medication, the anesthesiology team must share this information with the obstetrical team. It is equally important for the obstetrical team to alert the anesthesia team to the presence of bradycardia, so immediate preparations can be made for general anesthesia in the event regional anesthesia will not allow performing the C-section soon enough to avoid injuring the baby.

Should a complication occur, the first step toward correcting it is sharing knowledge of its existence with all members of the OB team. However, the obligation for good communication does not stop there. All members of the OB team must be informed of the steps being taken to correct the problem, as well as the success or failure of those steps, as they occur. Should the problem require emergency surgery, it should take place only after the mother is stabilized and the anesthesia team confirms she is ready.

Normally, a member of the anesthesia team meets with the mother before going to the OR. This meeting is the anesthesiologist's opportunity to ask questions about the mother's medical history and perform a physical examination (typically limited to the mouth, throat and the area of the spine where the anesthesia needle will be inserted) in case general anesthesia becomes necessary.

This meeting is also the mother's opportunity to question the anesthesiologist about the anesthesia and its side-effects, as well as to voice her expectations in the event of any complications, major or minor. The mother should be very clear that she expects the obstetrical team to be constantly informed, not only about how the administration of anesthesia is progressing, but also of any changes in her vital signs.

Finally, the mother should use this time to discuss who will be allowed in the operating room. The answer to this question is usually dictated by hospital policy or the obstetrician's and anesthesiologist's preferences. Normally, only one family member is permitted, but occasionally, two are allowed.

Remember, communication between the obstetrical and anesthesiology teams is critical, but communication between the family and each of these providers is equally important.

Hospital Policy

The hospital should have standing departmental policies requiring fetal monitoring in the operating room prior to C-section. Hospital policies also should provide for correct staffing and appropriate procedures for surgery preparation. Even if these policies are not in place, you can ensure the safety of both you and your baby by being well-informed, communicating specific expectations to your health care team, and getting their commitment to honor those requests.

Virtually all hospitals offer tours to expectant mothers. This tour provides a perfect opportunity to find out about the hospital's policies. It is also a good time to view the operating room and determine the type of fetal monitoring equipment that will be available during labor and delivery. Should the tour guide be unable to answer certain questions, do not hesitate to ask to speak to a nurse manager. They will almost always telephone you later, if you are unable to make contact at the time.

Additionally, during prenatal visits, ask your obstetrician about the hospital's policies. Be certain both you and your OB are fully informed.

Hospitals need your business to survive. Because their business is reputation-driven, they are not interested in practicing sub-par medicine. When doctors or patients raise issues, hospitals tend to take them very seriously. If you feel your concerns are not being met, you should address them with the hospital's administrative staff.

CHAPTER 4

Questions to Ask Your Obstetrician and Anesthesiologist

Well before you go to the hospital – and certainly before you go to the operating room – you should ask your health care team some important questions concerning regional anesthesia:

- Will steps be taken to confirm my well-being and that of my baby following administration of regional anesthesia?

- Will my obstetrician be present and ready to perform emergency surgery, if necessary?

- Who will be present in the OR and have direct responsibility for monitoring my vital signs?

- Who will be present in the OR and have direct responsibility for monitoring my baby's heart rate and well-being while I am under regional anesthesia?

- Will an electronic fetal monitor or a Doptone be in the operating room?

- Will I be advised of any complications that arise?

These questions reflect your awareness of the care you have a right to expect. Each question should be answered affirmatively. Your health care providers should not perceive the questions as antagonistic; it is your right and duty to safeguard your own health and that of your baby. These questions should be received in that spirit.

Make it clear to your obstetrician you require his or her presence not only for the delivery, but also during the administering of anesthesia.

If your health care providers' practices and plans do not meet the standards you expect, simply tell them your preferences and ask if they are acceptable. If not, that is the time to be politely assertive.

You should ask your obstetrician all these questions during prenatal care, well in advance of delivery. If that is not possible, ask them before you go to the operating room. If necessary, ask them when you are in the OR, before receiving regional anesthesia. Just be sure you ask them.

Make very sure, well in advance, that appropriate steps will be taken to ensure your safety and that of your baby. Don't assume anything. Your baby's future, as well as your own, depend on it.

PART III

Third-trimester Bleeding – When is it a Red Flag that Requires Hospitalization?

Getting to Know Your Placenta

Recognizing Uterine Rupture

CHAPTER 5

Diana's Story

Seven weeks shy of her due date, Diana awakens this Saturday morning to discover blood trickling from her vagina. Alarmed, she immediately calls her obstetrician's office and learns her doctor is not scheduled to work. The obstetrician covering for him soon returns Diana's call. She has never met this on-call doctor, but he seems to listen carefully and instructs her to go directly to the hospital.

Diana is admitted to the hospital at 8:40 a.m. The on-call doctor is not there. Thinking about their conversation, Diana realizes he didn't tell her when he would arrive.

At 9:15 a.m., yet another doctor Diana has never seen before enters the picture – the hospital's house obstetrician, who tells Diana he will manage her care until the on-call OB arrives.

Without examining Diana or inquiring about her prenatal care, the house doctor – relying on information from the attending obstetrical nurse – orders electronic fetal heart monitoring, injections of terbutaline (a medication to stop contractions), and an *immediate* fetal ultrasound. The objective of the emergency ultrasound is to rule out both placental abruption (premature separation of the placenta from the uterine wall) and placenta previa (abnormal positioning of the placenta at or near the internal opening of the cervix) as possible causes of the bleeding. Both of these conditions can be very dangerous to mother and baby.

At 9:40 a.m., the obstetrical nurse phones the radiology department to notify them the emergency ultrasound has been ordered. However, the radiology clerk mistakenly schedules it as a routine procedure. To make matters worse, no one on the OB team informs Diana about the need to perform the test immediately. The hospital staff keeps her completely in the dark.

At 10:30 a.m., the house obstetrician finally examines Diana and finds she is still bleeding. The ultrasound has not yet been performed, but the attending nurse has placed reminder call to radiology. This satisfies the house doctor, who leaves Diana to see another patient.

Although she does not know the fetal ultrasound was ordered on an expedited basis, after lying in the labor-and-delivery suite for nearly two hours, Diana begins to worry. *What is taking so long?*

So far, the baby's heart rate has been reassuring, but at 11:19 a.m., the attending nurse notices it has slowed somewhat. The on-call obstetrician still has not arrived, and the house OB is performing a C-section on another patient. With no doctor to consult, the nurse relies on her own interpretation of the EFM tracings. When the orderly arrives at 11:33 a.m. to transport Diana to radiology, the nurse gives the go-ahead, even though she is concerned about sending her to the basement, so far away from the labor-and-delivery suite.

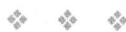

Now, Diana trembles as she lies under the thin sheet while a radiology technician performs the ultrasound. Her vaginal bleeding has increased. *Why didn't someone from the labor room come with me to monitor my baby?* She is terrified something has gone wrong with her little girl, whom she plans to name Julia. Diana has never felt so alone.

It is 11:42 a.m. The ultrasound registers a dangerously low fetal heart rate of only eighty-seven beats per minute – well below 110, the low end of the normal range. It also reveals the placenta has partially separated from the uterine wall – the extremely dangerous condition the house doctor suspected when he ordered the test. Even worse, the separation appears to be evolving. But instead of notifying the OB staff upstairs of the emergency unfolding and rushing Diana back upstairs, the technician takes the time to complete the analysis that is part of a routine ultrasound.

By the time the x-ray technician finishes, it is six minutes past noon. The baby's heart rate has dropped to sixty-eight beats per minute, yet the technician still does not notify the OB staff. Instead, she relays her findings to one of the staff radiologists, who merely prepares a report and sends it back to the OB floor with Diana.

At 12:45 p.m., the house obstetrician performs a second ultrasound at Diana's beside in her labor suite. He confirms the abruption, as well as the baby's precariously low heart rate. The house doctor then alerts the on-call physician, who orders an emergency C-section.

Although the on-call doctor – who sent Diana to the hospital more than four hours ago – has been at the hospital since a 12:15 p.m., he hasn't even checked on Diana He has left her care entirely to the house doctor.

At 1:47 p.m., a full hour after ordering an emergency C-section, the on-call doctor finally begins the procedure. Baby Julia is born at 1:52 p.m. She has suffered irreversible brain injuries consistent with a severe lack of oxygen shortly before birth.

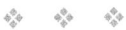

Today, Julia is a teenager. Despite the many challenges she and her mother confront when they wake each morning, they always seem to manage a smile. Diana finds comfort in believing Julia knows her parents love her with all their hearts. But Diana often cries herself to sleep at night, thinking about Julia's future – a future that won't include many of the joys experienced by healthy children and adults. Diana realizes her daughter will never act in a play or compete in sports. She will never go on a date or plan her wedding. She will never have children, but will always be childlike herself.

Knowing Julia's life didn't have to turn out this way only deepens Diana's sorrow. She feels betrayed by the doctors and hospital staff she entrusted with the birth of her precious daughter.

CHAPTER 6

What Went Wrong and Why

Introduction

Expectant mothers experience third-trimester vaginal bleeding in approximately six out of one hundred pregnancies. The causes and consequences of such bleeding range from inconsequential to severe. Even in very serious circumstances, permanent injury to the baby can often be prevented through timely recognition, appropriate corrective measures, and a speedy delivery, when necessary.

Diana's story focuses on one of the most troubling causes of third-trimester vaginal bleeding – placental abruption, or separation of the placenta from the uterine wall before birth. When placental abruption develops, the flow of oxygen and vital nutrients to the baby decreases or stops altogether. More than 30,000 incidents of placental abruption occur annually in the United States.

Failure to Properly Follow Up on Suspected Partial Abruption

A Potential Emergency

Diana's story involves a litany of missed opportunities and demonstrates how one bad decision can snowball, with life-altering consequences.

Virtually every member of the obstetrical team – the on-call obstetrician, the house doctor, the obstetrical nurses, the radiology technician, and the radiologist – mishandled Diana's and baby Julia's care.

The OB team allowed a potential obstetrical emergency, a partial abruption, to evolve into a profound catastrophe. They allowed Diana's placenta to continue separating prematurely from the uterine wall and her vaginal bleeding to increase, reducing the flow of blood (and oxygen) between mother and baby. This caused Julia's heart to slow dramatically, and eventually led to her brain damage.

Both the on-call obstetrician and the house obstetrician suspected a partial abruption, but they dropped the ball when it came time to conscientiously following up – even after the abruption was verified and Julia's dangerously slow heart rate was discovered.

Had the obstetricians, obstetrical nurse, radiology staff, and those responsible for establishing safe procedures at the hospital met applicable standards of care, the events of Julia's birth would have played out very differently.

Zone of Safety

Once a partial abruption is suspected, especially one with ongoing vaginal bleeding, the condition should be treated as an emergency until proven otherwise. An immediate C-section may be necessary to save the mother's life, prevent a debilitating birth injury to the baby, or both. That means keeping the expectant mother in the labor-and-delivery suite – the *zone of safety* – where operating rooms are located, and necessary obstetrical and anesthesia staff can be quickly assembled.

If vaginal bleeding has ceased for twenty-four consecutive hours and the fetal heart rate is thoroughly reassuring, consideration may then be given to moving the expectant mother to the obstetrical high-risk ward.

Bedside Ultrasound

With a working diagnosis of placental abruption, an expectant mother should be fully evaluated within the zone of safety the obstetrical suite provides. A properly equipped and staffed obstetrical department should be able to quickly verify a suspected abruption. Basic ultrasound machinery is all that is necessary.

The hospital had the equipment and personnel to perform Diana's ultrasound in the labor-and-delivery suite. However, the obstetrical staff sent her down to the basement, where the radiology department was located. Just as the in-house obstetrician performed the second ultrasound at Diana's bedside in the labor-and-delivery suite, the first ultrasound should have been performed there. The failure to do so after a working diagnosis of placental abruption clearly breached the standard of care.

With a bedside ultrasound, Diana's test results would have been available to the OB staff immediately. Her partial abruption would have been detected sooner, before Julia's heart rate slowed and while mother and baby were still safely in the labor-and-delivery suite.

The house doctor started down the right path when he ordered an immediate ultrasound, but he took a wrong turn when he chose not to perform the ultrasound on the spot.

Continuous EFM

The attending obstetrical nurse compounded the mistake of authorizing the orderly to transport Diana to radiology by failing to accompany Diana in order to constantly monitor the fetal heart rate on the way to radiology, while Diana was awaiting the ultrasound, and during the return trip. Julia was completely unmonitored during these critical periods.

The house obstetrician appropriately ordered electronic fetal heart monitoring, but failed to specify EFM was to be maintained continuously. That omission left room for the attending nurse to misinterpret his order.

In circumstances like Diana's, where a suspected partial abruption has not stabilized, uninterrupted EFM must be maintained until vaginal bleeding has ceased for at least twenty-four hours, and fetal heart rate tracings are completely reassuring.

Obstetrician Should Have Interpreted Tracings

The attending obstetrical nurse missed still another opportunity to keep Diana in the labor-and-delivery suite. Before disconnecting the EFM just prior to transporting Diana to radiology, she observed the EFM tracings had revealed a troubling drop in Julia's heart rate. This non-reassuring fetal heart pattern gave the nurse second thoughts about sending Diana downstairs, but she sent her anyway, without first alerting the house obstetrician to the change in Julia's condition and getting his input.

The obstetrical nurse had an explanation: she thought her actions were justified because an obstetrician was not immediately available to interpret the fetal monitor printout. She thought wrong.

This nursing error deprived Diana and her baby of the crucial benefit of having an obstetrician analyze vital EFM data. Diana's nurse should have torn off at least fifteen minutes' worth of the tracings and taken them into the operating room where the house obstetrician was performing a C-section. As soon as circumstances permitted, he could have evaluated the tracings and issued appropriate orders right there in the OR. An obstetrician is expected to multi-task under such circumstances. Appropriate orders would have included an immediate bedside ultrasound while preparations began for an emergency C-section.

Communication and Other Basic Breakdowns

Diana and Julia were victims of breakdowns in even rudimentary aspects of obstetrical care.

The communication gaffe between the obstetrical nurse and the radiology clerk resulted in the clerk's scheduling the ultrasound as a routine procedure, exponentially increasing the delay and risk of performing Diana's ultrasound in radiology, rather than in the labor-and-delivery suite. There is no room for sloppy communication in obstetrics or any field of health care.

Both the obstetrical nurse and the house doctor knew Diana's transport to radiology was delayed, but they failed to find out why. Had they investigated, they would have learned the ultrasound had been mistakenly scheduled as routine. This error would have been corrected, and valuable hours would have been saved.

What to Expect from an On-Call Obstetrician

Where was the on-call obstetrician who was covering for Diana's private physician while all this was unfolding?

First, he took his time getting to the hospital. Once there, he was slow to check on the patient he had sent directly to the hospital hours earlier – a patient he had never seen before and whose medical history he did not know. He had every reason to suspect Diana was facing a potential obstetrical emergency, yet he did not provide her with the timely bedside management of her condition she expected and deserved.

In essence, the on-call OB treated Diana like a second-class citizen, sloughing off primary responsibility for her care to the hospital's in-house obstetrician. Would he have treated one of his own patients that way? The on-call physician should have provided Diana and Julia with the same attention and quality of care he would give one of his own patients. Anything less is unacceptable.

What to Expect from a House Obstetrician

Typically, the responsibilities of the house obstetrician include evaluating patients as quickly as circumstances dictate after they arrive on the obstetrical floor, treating patients who do not have private doctors, and dealing with emergencies. The house OB may confer with a private obstetrician regarding the patient's status to ascertain whether the private physician's presence is necessary.

If the on-call OB or the patient's regular physician negligently exposes the patient to a significant risk of injury, the house obstetrician is expected to intervene. That obligation is imposed only if the house doctor knew, or should have known, about the deficiency in care and was available to help. The on-call obstetrician, not the house OB, is primarily responsible for the patient's care.

On this busy Saturday, the in-house obstetrician did himself and Donna a grave disservice by not insisting the on-call doctor come to the hospital to attend to his patient; the need for his presence was clear. The house obstetrician was managing the care of several other patients, including preparing to perform a C-section on one. However, instead of summoning the on-call obstetrician, the house OB allowed himself to be taken advantage of, seriously jeopardizing Diana's and Julia's well-being.

Hospital Policies and Protocols

To ensure proper obstetrical care for patients admitted with a possible abruption, hospital officials are expected to have safe, standardized operating procedures in place. But that's not enough. They also must take steps to ensure those protocols are followed by all hospital staff and physicians with practicing privileges in the hospital.

Not a single member of Diana's heath care team appeared to know Diana should be kept in the zone of safety and her baby needed continuous fetal monitoring. Appropriate, strictly enforced hospital policies would have ensured Diana remained in the labor-and-delivery suite, with her baby undergoing continuous electronic fetal heart monitoring.

Failure to Inform the Expectant Mother

Diana was kept out of the loop entirely. No one informed her about the need to verify her condition quickly or the possibility of an emergency C-section. She was left to either rely on intuition or call upon information she had acquired on her own. Eventually, Diana's intuition kicked in, but she didn't have the knowledge to be certain her concerns were valid, and she didn't understand time was of the essence.

Diana relied 100 percent on her doctor's knowledge and reliability to attend closely to her needs during labor and delivery. She did not educate herself independently, in advance of delivery, about how health care providers should handle a potential obstetrical complication such as a suspected placental abruption.

Failure to Respond Appropriately to a Known Partial Abruption and Fetal Bradycardia

A Confirmed Emergency

It's one thing to fail to respond properly to a suspected emergency; it's another thing entirely to fail to respond to a confirmed, known emergency. In this case, hospital personnel observed an evolving placental abruption and a sustained, severe drop in fetal heart rate. Yet, they continued to subject Diana and her baby to further lapses in care. As the potential emergency ripened into a frightening reality, hospital personnel continued a pattern of indifference toward both patients' health and safety.

Radiology

Ultrasound technicians should be acutely aware an abruption of recent origin may signal a true medical emergency, posing grave risks for the mother and the baby, in particular. They should be equally aware that, after they confirm both the presence of an acute abruption and a persistently low fetal heart rate via ultrasound, there is no

longer any doubt that an emergency exists. The presence of ongoing vaginal bleeding is not required to validate it, although Diana
not only continued to bleed, but the flow of vaginal blood actually
increased.

After an emergency of this nature is confirmed, it no longer matters whether an ultrasound was ordered routinely or emergently. The
ultrasound procedure should be ceased and a member of the patient's
obstetrical team notified immediately. In a hospital setting, the patient should be returned to the labor-and-delivery suite immediately
and an emergency C-section performed without delay.

The radiology technician performing Diana's ultrasound observed
the abruption and low fetal heart rate. Apparently oblivious to the
gravity of the situation, she notified no one and continued to take and
evaluate images. She checked Julia's bone length, head size and body
weight, and methodically went through the rest of the steps associated
with a routine ultrasound for a baby of her gestational age.

The radiologist who arrived to interpret the ultrasound images also
proceeded on a business-as-usual basis. In violation of the most minimal standard of care, he simply entered the red-flag findings on Diana's
chart and took no steps to alert anyone about the emergency at hand.

Back on the Obstetrical Floor

Eventually, Diana was returned to her labor-and-delivery suite,
along with her hospital chart. Although the radiology report contained all the evidence he needed, the house OB performed a repeat
ultrasound at Diana's bedside. Again, the results verified the diagnosis
he initially suspected – a placental abruption.

By that time, every minute counted. Incredibly, Julia's delivery
was still delayed. None of the evidence seemed to light a fire under
anyone – not firsthand observation of the evolving abruption, not the
ultrasound results, not the dangerously low fetal heart rate, and not
Diana's increased vaginal bleeding.

The evidence did prompt the house obstetrician to telephone the on-call OB, who was elsewhere in the hospital. After conferring, they decided to wait for the on-call OB to perform Diana's C-section. When further delay should have been unthinkable, another hour was wasted as a result of that fateful decision.

What should the house doctor have done instead? He should have called for anesthesia on an emergency basis, cut into Diana's abdomen and delivered Julia within a few minutes. At that point, every minute Julia remained in her mother's womb meant another minute without oxygen and more extensive brain injury.

CHAPTER 7

What Expectant Mothers Should Know

Time Frame and Bleeding Sites

The third trimester starts in the twenty-eighth week or seventh month of pregnancy. Bleeding that develops during this time frame is generally found at the site of the vagina, urethra or rectum. Whatever the apparent source of the bleeding, you should immediately notify your obstetrician, who then can evaluate the circumstances and determine the extent of risk. In many cases, it is necessary to go directly to the hospital for an immediate, thorough examination because the source of the vaginal bleeding may be a more internal part of the body, as with Diana.

Degrees of Bleeding

The amount of blood can vary, from spotting to a single gush or a continuous flow. A continuous flow may be light to very heavy. With the exception of heavy bleeding, third-trimester bleeding often resolves without incident. Even if you are experiencing only light vaginal bleeding, however, you should take the condition seriously, as should your obstetrician.

Placental Abruption

Functions of the Placenta

The placenta is a temporary organ that serves both baby and mother during pregnancy. About the size of a deflated soccer ball at term, the placenta develops inside the uterus, along with the baby. The placenta allows the mother's blood, which contains oxygen and nutrients, to flow from the mother to the fetus, and deoxygenated blood and waste products to flow from the fetus to the mother.

How is this accomplished? The mother's blood travels to the uterus and flows into her side of the placenta where many substances in the blood, such as certain medications, bacteria, viruses and maternal antibodies are filtered and substantially blocked from reaching the baby. The umbilical cord, which contains blood vessels and extends into the baby's side of the placenta, carries freshly oxygenated blood from the placenta to the baby. A separate vessel within the cord carries blood that has already circulated through the baby's body, and therefore contains waste products, back to the baby's side of the placenta. The waste products pass into the mother's blood supply and ultimately are disposed of through her kidneys. When the placenta is functioning properly, the mother's blood and the baby's blood, which may be of different types, do not mix.

In order for the baby to receive sufficient oxygen and nourishment, and develop properly, the placenta must remain attached to the uterine wall throughout pregnancy.

Normally, the placenta is expelled following delivery. You may have heard the placenta referred to as the "afterbirth."

Risk Factors and Causes

The most predictive risk factor of abruption is a history of abruption in a previous pregnancy. It is imperative to inform your obstetrician if you have such a history.

Other risk factors include advanced maternal age; multiple previous births; multiple fetuses in a single pregnancy, such as twins; blood clotting disorders; high blood pressure; preeclampsia, which is a dangerous combination in the mother of increased blood pressure, excessive protein in the urine, and marked swelling of the extremities and face; premature rupture of membranes, which is deemed to occur when water breaks before the onset of contractions; an abnormally high amount of amniotic fluid; the presence of uterine fibroids; smoking cigarettes; and cocaine use.

Trauma to the abdomen may also cause an abruption. This can occur in any number of ways, from falling forward to the sudden tightening of the seat belt in a car accident. Any kind of trauma to the abdomen should be reported to the obstetrician immediately, and the fetus should be monitored with an external fetal monitor for at least six hours afterward.

During the third trimester, the baby and placenta grow more rapidly than at any other time, approximately tripling in size. While abruptions can occur earlier in pregnancy, the risk of abruption is greatest during this period of accelerated growth.

Signs and Symptoms of Abruption

The most common symptoms of abruption are vaginal bleeding and abdominal pain, but an abruption does not always produce vaginal bleeding. In some cases, a blood clot may form between the placenta and the uterine wall, or there may be no visible sign of bleeding at all. If an abruption develops without visible bleeding, it is known as an *occult* or *silent* abruption.

An abruption not signaled by vaginal bleeding is potentially more challenging to diagnose, but it is by no means undetectable. Indeed, it is relatively simple to determine whether occult bleeding has occurred. A blood test that includes evaluating the mother's hematocrit value (the percentage of red blood cells in a sample of blood) usually evidences any recent blood loss. Another blood test called a *Kleihauer-Betcke (KB) test* can detect the presence of fetal red blood cells in the mother's blood. A positive result confirms an abruption has occurred. Further, an abdominal ultrasound is just as capable of revealing a silent abruption as one that produces vaginal bleeding.

Whether bleeding is present or not, with the exception of particularly small abruptions that may avoid detection, partial and total abruptions are usually detectable via ultrasound. However, failure to visualize an abruption on ultrasound does not rule out its presence.

Abdominal pain associated with an abruption sometimes manifests itself in the form of tetanic contractions. These contractions feel like severe muscle spasms, similar to an extremely painful charley horse, and the uterus does not relax as it normally would between contractions. The symptoms of abdominal pain and bleeding that signal abruption normally begin rather suddenly, but a slow onset with increasing intensity is also possible.

Placental abruption can also be indicated by other symptoms. You may experience uterine hyper-stimulation–contractions that occur in quick succession, with little or no break between them. Additionally, specific types of fetal heart rate patterns may suggest an abruption. Two examples are persistent drops below 110 beats per minute that fail to return to normal until well after each contraction has concluded and unrelenting bradycardia. In some cases, further investigation is appropriate; in others, immediate delivery is mandatory.

Acute Abruption versus Chronic Abruption
Abruptions are classified either as *acute* (an abruption of recent onset) or *chronic* (an abruption of longer duration that has stabilized).

When the placenta first begins to separate from the uterus, the abruption is acute. An acute total abruption or near-total abruption always constitutes an emergency. A less severe acute partial abruption can also require emergency intervention. The status of the baby, as determined by electronic fetal heart monitoring, is key. If the EFM tracings do not reliably assure the baby's well-being, immediate action is mandatory.

When time clearly permits, ultrasound technology may be used to perform a biophysical profile for a more extensive assessment of fetal well-being. This testing is accompanied by electronic fetal heart monitoring and goes far beyond ascertaining whether an abruption is present. It includes evaluation of four additional measures of fetal health – amniotic fluid volume, fetal breathing movement, fetal tone, and fetal gross body movements.

Some acute abruptions stabilize and enter a chronic phase. The requirements for reclassification are no further bleeding; no further separation of the placenta from the uterine wall; and twenty-four continuous hours of fetal well-being, which must be documented by EFM tracings. A stabilized abruption poses a lesser, more manageable risk to mother and baby.

It is possible a small amount of dark, red blood may continue to pass for several days after an abruption has stabilized. Even after an abruption has become chronic, the placenta can separate from the uterus, once again becoming acute. While mild abruptions frequently stabilize, moderate and severe abruptions usually do not.

Risks Associated with Placental Abruption

Risks to Baby

If blood flow between the uterus and placenta decreases greatly and delivery is not accomplished right away, the baby is at risk of suffering permanent brain damage or death. A well-oxygenated and otherwise-healthy baby may tolerate a near-total abruption for about ten to fifteen minutes before the onset of permanent damage.

If only a mild or moderate partial abruption has occurred, the baby may tolerate the deficient environment for a longer period. How long the baby withstands these circumstances varies with the extent and duration of the abruption, and the baby's oxygen reserves (the level of the baby's oxygenation before the abruption occurred).

Performing an emergency delivery in the case of abruption frequently avoids permanent injury to the baby due to lack of oxygen. However, if such a delivery is forced with a premature baby, birth injury stemming from prematurity itself is possible. Very young babies whose vital organs are not sufficiently developed are vulnerable to brain injury, cerebral palsy, and death. Medical advancements that help even very small preemies survive do not rule out the possibility of permanent harm from prematurity.

Finally, the loss of blood as a result of abruption can also cause varying degrees of anemia in the baby.

Risks to Mother

Placental abruptions can have life-threatening implications for mothers, with blood loss being the primary cause. These risks range from mild anemia to organ damage and even death. Severe, permanent harm to mothers is rare. Mothers have a greater ability than babies to tolerate the amount of blood loss ordinarily associated with even a significant abruption, and they directly benefit from stabilizing medical support, such as blood transfusion and volume replacement. Conversely, doctors have no direct access to the baby until after delivery and must provide all therapies indirectly, through the mother.

When Complications Arise

Corrective Measures for Baby

A near-total or complete abruption requires immediate delivery. In the case of a near-term or full-term baby, permanent fetal injury often can be avoided with timely delivery. If the abruption occurs when mother does not have access to immediate medical attention, the likelihood of a good outcome for the baby is reduced.

If an abruption necessitating delivery develops early in the pregnancy, the outcome depends not only on a timely delivery, but also on the baby's gestational age and development. In a case of partial abruption not requiring immediate delivery, therapies are available to speed up the baby's maturing process. A primary component of this therapy is giving medication to speed up lung development, so the baby can breathe more efficiently.

Regardless of whether emergency surgery is required, steps should be taken to maximize the flow of blood and oxygen to the baby. Many of the corrective measures for the mother explained below indirectly help achieve these objectives. For instance, restricting her to bed rest and administering oxygen and fluids are among the most helpful actions. Another effective measure is turning her on her side to alleviate pressure on her great vessels and allow blood to flow more freely to the uterus and the baby.

After delivery, when the pediatric team has direct access to the baby, numerous resuscitative measures are available. If delivery is timely, the infant may require only stimulation and oxygen; however, if the baby's condition is critical, full "code" procedures may be necessary. These procedures may include intubation (inserting a breathing tube into the trachea to deliver oxygen to the lungs efficiently), cardiopulmonary resuscitation (CPR), or administration of intravenous fluids and medication.

Corrective Measures for Mother

When placental abruption results in profuse bleeding, waiting for a natural vaginal delivery of the baby and placenta is not an option. Under these circumstances, it is imperative to attempt to stop the bleeding by performing an immediate Caesarean section and removing the placenta.

A blood transfusion may also be necessary. To prepare for this possibility, as your delivery time nears, you should have a sample of your blood sent to the hospital's blood bank. At the very least, the hospital should compare your blood type to the blood they have in storage, ensuring the availability of a safe transfusion.

Usually, an anesthesiologist orders and oversees a blood transfusion. The anesthesiologist also performs supportive measures, such as starting an IV to allow blood and fluids to be administered quickly, and administering medications to help the mother's heart pump efficiently and maintain an adequate blood flow throughout her body.

On the rare occasions when uterine bleeding cannot be stopped, an emergency hysterectomy must be performed. This is done only as a lifesaving procedure and only after the surgeon has exhausted all other surgical interventions.

When vaginal bleeding does not require emergency intervention, careful observation of mother and baby is acceptable. Two to three additional days of close observation in a high-risk pregnancy unit are appropriate, followed by discharge to home with instructions to remain primarily on bed rest. Observation should take place in the labor-and-delivery suite until active bleeding has stopped.

Finally, third-trimester bleeding due to abruption, and the abruption itself, can be worsened by uterine contractions. If the baby is preterm (less than thirty-six to thirty-seven weeks) and emergency surgical delivery is not required, attempts should be made to stop the contractions. If the contractions lessen, bleeding usually subsides. Even in this circumstance, though, it may be necessary for mother to remain on medication to suppress contractions until the baby reaches term.

Placenta Previa

Placenta previa occurs when the placenta covers all or part of the internal opening of the cervix, known as the *internal cervical os*. If the os is totally covered, the previa is deemed to be total. If only a portion of the os is covered, the condition is referred to as a *partial previa*, and is depicted in this illustration (FIG. 1).

POSITION OF PLACENTA (FIG. 1)

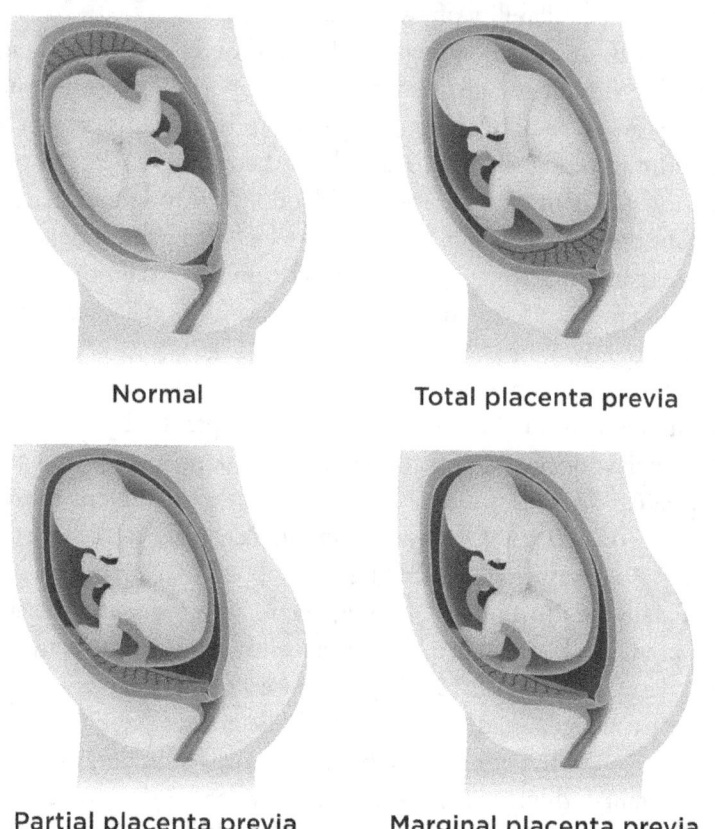

Normal   Total placenta previa

Partial placenta previa   Marginal placenta previa

The placenta is a pancake-shaped organ that normally attaches itself to the uterine wall, away from the cervical opening. It can be located on the anterior, posterior or lateral wall of the uterus. It can also be attached at the top of the uterus, as shown here. This is called a *fundal* location. Occasionally, the placenta implants on the lower uterine wall; in this instance, if any part of the placenta is involved with the cervical opening, it is called a *placenta previa*. The three types of previa get their names from the extent of involvement with the cervix and are depicted in this diagram.

The majority of placenta previas are diagnosed during routine second-trimester ultrasounds. However, bleeding associated with previa does not ordinarily occur until the third trimester, following the onset of contractions.

In cases of placenta previa, the placenta not only covers all or part of the cervix, it is actually attached to part of the cervix. The placenta tears when the cervix begins to dilate during labor. Bleeding quickly follows, as does a reduction in the flow of blood to the baby. For these reasons, labor and vaginal delivery almost always must be avoided.

Any activity that can bring on contractions and cervical dilation should also be avoided. This includes sexual activity such as intercourse, clitoral stimulation, and even nipple stimulation, which can cause your body to release oxytocin, a substance that makes your uterus contract. Dehydration should be guarded against and exercise curtailed. Finally, mothers with previa should avoid pelvic examinations, which can cause tearing of the placenta.

Vaginal bleeding is often the first sign of previa. Bleeding associated with previa is usually fairly brisk, bright red in color and painless. The absence of pain differentiates a placenta previa from other serious causes of third-trimester bleeding.

Once uncontrolled bleeding develops in the third trimester as a result of placenta previa, the diagnostic and treatment measures for mother and baby are virtually the same as those that apply to abruption. If you are at or near term, delivery by C-section should be undertaken expeditiously. If you are early in your pregnancy, management options depend on the amount of bleeding, the stability of your vital signs, and the well-being of your baby.

It is impossible to predict with certainty the timing and severity of when bleeding will occur. In the presence of a known previa, your hematocrit should be monitored as a precaution. If it slips below thirty, remedial steps such as an iron supplement should be taken. In some cases, a blood transfusion may be needed.

Time permitting, the baby's well-being should be determined by performing a biophysical profile and a non-stress test. Careful, continuous fetal observation can be done as an alternative, as long as the baby maintains reassuring EFM tracings. All of these evaluations and therapies should be carried out within the zone of safety, the labor-and-delivery suite. If bleeding becomes profuse or the baby's status ceases to be reassuring, emergency delivery is mandatory.

A previa diagnosed early in the pregnancy may self-correct. If uterine growth causes the placenta to migrate up the uterine wall and off the cervical opening, placenta previa ceases to be an impediment to vaginal delivery. Periodic ultrasound examinations should be conducted to verify the location of the placenta and determine whether a safe vaginal delivery is once again possible. Even if placenta previa no longer appears to be a concern, when you arrive at the hospital for delivery, always alert your obstetrical team that a previa was identified earlier in your pregnancy.

Uterine Rupture

In addition to abruption and placenta previa, uterine rupture represents another potentially dangerous cause of third-trimester bleeding. Differentiating between the three is important and can often be done with a thorough patient history.

Uterine rupture occurs almost exclusively in women who have had prior uterine surgery. Examples include C-sections, removal of fibroid tumors (myomectomy), repair of uterine perforation during a D&C or an abortion, and reconstruction of the uterus to resolve fertility issues.

It is important to notify your obstetrician of any surgical procedures you have undergone that involved the uterus, no matter how trivial they may seem. Your doctor should obtain the operative notes to aid in making an informed recommendation about whether labor is safe and advisable.

Bleeding from uterine rupture is usually profuse. The most common presentation of uterine rupture – even more so than uterine bleeding – is searing or burning pain across the lower abdomen. Usually, the pain is continuous, even in the absence of or between contractions. Pain that has these characteristics is different from the type associated with abruption. Obviously, you should report pain of this or any type to your obstetrical team immediately. It is particularly important to report any changes in the character of your pain.

Another possible symptom of uterine rupture is shoulder pain. This is caused by blood in the abdominal cavity irritating the nerves in the diaphragm that carry sensation to the shoulder.

Unrelenting, non-reassuring fetal heart rate patterns will eventually develop with uterine rupture, and when they do, emergency surgery is required. However, it would be extremely dangerous to wait for a persistent drop in the fetal heart rate before diagnosing a potential rupture and intervening surgically. Surgical intervention should be initiated in response to the other signs and symptoms of uterine rupture, which often occur before any effects on the fetal heart rate are notable.

Of the three causes of third-trimester bleeding on which we have focused, uterine rupture is the only one that always requires emergency surgery. Without surgery, neither mother nor baby can be expected to survive.

Although uterine rupture is relatively rare, when it does occur, the risks of a devastating outcome are great. If you have had prior uterine surgery, it is imperative you have an in-depth discussion with your obstetrician regarding the risks of labor, including the speed with which surgery must be performed to avoid severe fetal injury. Without this information, you cannot make an informed decision about whether to undergo labor in the hope of delivering vaginally, or to forgo labor and have a repeat C-section. If you decide to attempt vaginal delivery, you and your entire obstetrical team – including the doctor who may be covering for your obstetrician – should be fully prepared to coordinate an emergency delivery if one becomes necessary.

Benign Causes of Third-Trimester Bleeding

Fortunately, third-trimester bleeding usually emanates from the portion of the cervix that rests in the vagina and is not harmful to mother or baby. During pregnancy, the blood vessels in this segment of the cervix become extremely engorged (swollen), somewhat sensitive, and easily broken. Even light touch to this area can cause bleeding. Intercourse and pelvic exams are the two most common causes of this type of third-trimester bleeding, which is usually painless and produces a bright red flow.

This section of the cervix is also extremely sensitive to bacterial infection. The vagina normally contains a variety of bacteria. These bacteria may cause cervicitis, a localized infection in the vaginal part of the cervix. This rarely puts the baby at risk, but it can cause spotting.

Sexually transmitted diseases, such as trichomonas and chlamydia, may also cause cervicitis and spotting. Although the bleeding caused by these types of infections is not harmful, if left untreated, they may cause other problems, such as preterm labor.

Urinary tract infections also occur frequently during pregnancy. The most serious infections may cause some bleeding in the urethra and bladder. When this occurs, spotting may appear on toilet tissue when cleansing after urination. This virtually never affects the baby. It is important to identify any infectious agent and treat it with appropriate medication.

Nearly all expectant mothers develop hemorrhoids to some degree during the third trimester as a result of engorgement of blood vessels in the rectal area. Occasionally, hemorrhoids bleed, sometimes quite heavily, due to straining with or without a bowel movement. Because of the large abdominal distention during the third trimester, expectant mothers are sometimes unable to definitively determine whether the source of bleeding is vaginal or anal.

Whenever third-trimester bleeding develops, don't hesitate to contact the obstetrician overseeing your pregnancy. Often, the cause can be determined over the telephone with a thorough review of your relevant medical history and the current situation. If it is necessary for you to be examined, don't delay the exam or allow your physician to delay it. If there is uncertainty about the seriousness of your bleeding, you and your doctor should err on the side of caution, and you should be seen and evaluated in the hospital's obstetrical department on an emergency basis.

CHAPTER 8

Questions to Ask Your Obstetrician

Before you go to the hospital, ask these important questions of your obstetrician and health care team:

- If I develop third-trimester vaginal bleeding and placenta abruption, uterine rupture, or placenta previa are suspected, will I be informed?

- Will I be examined and thoroughly evaluated for these conditions within an hour of my arrival at the hospital or sooner, if circumstances warrant?

- Will ultrasound equipment be available bedside in the labor-and-delivery suite, eliminating the need to transport me out of the zone of safety if this diagnostic test becomes necessary?

- If it becomes necessary to transport me to radiology or another department, will a nurse trained in electronic fetal heart monitoring accompany me and monitor my baby's well-being continuously?

- If an EFM tracing reveals a persistent non-reassuring fetal heart rate pattern, will the tracing be analyzed immediately by an obstetrician, rather than an obstetrical nurse?

- Will the anesthesia staff and other operating room personnel be immediately available if an emergency C-section becomes necessary?

- Will an experienced pediatric team be present at delivery if there is reason for concern about my baby's well-being?

- If an on-call physician is responsible for my obstetrical care, will I receive the same attention and quality of care I expect from my regular physician?

PART IV

Inducing Labor – Don't Get Hyper About It

Keeping Tabs on Your Contractions and Baby with Electronic Fetal Monitoring

Your Placenta Revisited

CHAPTER 9

Alexandra's Story

On a snowy Friday evening, Alexandra sits anxiously in the passenger seat of the family car. Her husband is carefully maneuvering their rear-wheel-drive vehicle over slippery roads. But it's not the weather, the road conditions, or the absence of four-wheel drive that is causing her concern. It's the purpose of the trip. She's heading to the labor-and-delivery department of a university hospital to have labor induced – *three weeks before her due date.*

Alex's obstetrician doesn't want to wait for the pregnancy to run its natural course. He doesn't even want to wait until the weekend is over – although it means she and her husband must brave a storm to get to the hospital. *This can't be good,* Alex thinks. *Please, please don't let anything bad happen to my baby.*

A below-normal level of amniotic fluid, a condition known as *oligohydramnios,* has been present on and off for three months. It has become more significant lately. Making matters worse, two days ago, Alex detected decreased fetal movement, although it improved after lying on her left side for an hour. This evening, just after dinner, Alex again sensed her baby was much less active than usual. She immediately alerted her obstetrician. That's when he decided to speed up the timetable for delivery.

The confluence of these complications raised doubt in Alex's doctor's mind about her baby's ability to safely remain in her womb much longer. His biggest concern is that the placenta, which babies depend on for oxygen and nutrition during pregnancy, might be wearing out prematurely.

Alex arrives at the hospital and completes her admission paperwork by 8:30 p.m. Within fifteen minutes, she settles into the labor-and-delivery suite, and an obstetrical nurse performs a limited vaginal examination. Alex's cervix is one centimeter dilated, and the membranes holding in the amniotic fluid are intact. Labor and vaginal delivery will not occur naturally any time soon.

Next, the nurse wraps a belt with a built-in sensor around Alex's abdomen, connecting her to an electronic fetal monitoring device. The device provides vital information about the fetus' well-being via heart rate tracings. Unborn babies communicate with the outside world about their health through these tracings. The monitor also records Alex's contraction pattern below her baby's heart tracing.

Alex is somewhat familiar with the process. She has been hooked up to EFM equipment several times in recent months because of her low amniotic fluid. But Alex has no idea what the different fetal heart patterns mean. No obstetrician or obstetrical nurse has ever taken the initiative to explain them to her, and they were only mentioned superficially in her birthing class. Nor does this first-time mother in her early twenties think she needs to know about them. Alex relies completely on her obstetrical team to interpret what her baby's heart is saying. Up to this point, her lack of knowledge – even about the right questions to ask – hasn't mattered.

Alex stares at tray that will catch the graph paper as it cascades out of the EFM equipment. Her apprehension intensifies. While she waits for the tracings and their translation, she bites down hard on her lower lip.

Moments later, a graph bearing a pattern that resembles a zigzag shape, like the teeth of a saw, lands in the tray. The tracing shows

Alex's baby's heart rate consistently fluctuating in the range of 130-140 beats per minute. After studying the tracings intently, the doctor determines an emergency C-section isn't warranted, and they can try to induce labor instead.

Alex is relieved, not only that her baby is healthy, but also that she can deliver vaginally. Soon, she begins to see the bright side of delivering three weeks early. *I'll have Nick Jr. in my arms three weeks sooner. And hopefully, I'll be back to a size six that much sooner.*

The process of inducing labor begins. First, the nurse places a medication called *Cytotec* (misoprostol) to the back of the vagina near Alex's cervix, the neck-like, constricted lower end of the uterus. The medication works by thinning out (effacing) the cervix and causing contractions in an effort to advance the labor process.

Cytotec is applied by Alex's cervix three times, but progress is slow and arduous. At about 5:40 p.m. on Saturday, nearly twenty-one hours after induction was begun, Alex's OB directs the nursing staff to move on to the next induction drug, an intravenously administered drug called *Pitocin*. Often used after Cytotec begins the labor process, Pitocin mimics a natural substance the body secretes to induce contractions strong enough to bring about the cervical changes necessary to deliver vaginally. Once the cervix is dilated to ten centimeters and 100 percent effaced (fully thinned out), Alex will be able to start pushing.

The Pitocin induces contractions that increase in frequency and intensity over time – as they should, but within limits. By about 3:00 a.m. Sunday, roughly thirty hours after induction began, Alex's water breaks. A sterile vaginal exam (SVE) reveals her cervix has dilated one more centimeter, for a total of two, and she is 70 percent effaced. Alex's son has taken his first baby step into the birth canal. In clinical terms related to his positioning, baby Nick has reached -2 station, with +5 station being the final destination, just before delivery. Labor is progressing, although it is still in the very early stages.

With Alex's labor spanning such a long period of time, hospital personnel shifts occur. Her nurses, resident physicians, and even her private physician who directed her to come to the hospital, all go home and are replaced by an entirely new obstetrical team. These changes in staff increase the importance of seamless communication between those who have been caring for Alex and baby Nick, and those who are assuming their care.

At about 6:00 a.m., thirty-three hours into the induction process, another SVE is performed. Alex's cervix is now three and one-half centimeters dilated and 100 percent effaced. Baby Nick has moved a bit farther into the birth canal, to -1 station.

Intermittently since 4:00 a.m., hospital personnel have noted some fleeting minor fetal heart rate decelerations. Each time, the heart rate resolved on its own. Now, shortly after 7:00 a.m., new and potentially more significant fetal heart rate changes begin to appear and are not improving. In fact, the fetal heart rate is slowing with almost every contraction. For the first time in Alex's labor, the EFM tracings are not reassuring of baby Nick's well-being. Essentially, he is calling out from the uterus, asking for help in the only way he can.

The nurse caring for Alex heeds her baby's distress calls and quickly initiates intrauterine resuscitative measures (IURM). First, she positions Alex on her side to take pressure off the vena cava, a large vein situated next to the spine, which increases the flow of blood to Alex's heart. Alex's blood is then pumped to her lungs, where waste products her blood is carrying are exchanged for oxygen. The freshly oxygenated blood then travels back to Alex's heart before it flows on to the baby. Second, she gives Alex oxygen by mask to increase the amount of oxygen available to her baby. Next, she administers a large-scale infusion (bolus) of intravenous fluids to Alex to further help increase the flow of oxygenated blood to baby Nick. Finally, the nurse decreases the dosage of Pitocin in order to slow and weaken Alex's contractions, thereby reducing stress on the baby.

But the non-reassuring EFM tracings persist. The efforts to rejuvenate baby Nick don't appear to be working. And another finding is even more troubling – the deterioration in a fetal heart rate parameter called *variability*, which measures variation or fluctuation of the baby's heart rate on a beat-to-beat or more long-term basis.

Intrauterine resuscitative measures do not always adequately resuscitate the baby, but they are often effective. When they are, the results are usually apparent within five to ten minutes of initiation. In Alex's case, they take a bit longer. Approximately fifteen minutes elapse before her baby's heart rate decelerations disappear from the tracings, indicating he is satisfactorily oxygenated, at least for the moment. As a precaution, the nurse consults a resident physician. Both are satisfied that the induction of labor can continue, so they increase the dosage of Pitocin to the amount that was originally ordered.

However, it is not long before the non-reassuring fetal heart rate patterns reappear. Several more times, the tracings signal periods of significantly decreased oxygen being delivered to the baby. Each time, it takes longer for him to recuperate following administration of IURM. Each time, it takes a toll on baby Nick's capacity to withstand the stress of labor and vaginal delivery. And each time, the physician and nursing staff conclude it is safe to continue inducing labor and resume the dose of Pitocin that contributed to recurrent non-reassuring fetal heart rate patterns.

Eventually, Alex and her husband suspect something is wrong and begin asking questions. The nurse provides a cursory explanation of the tracings, downplaying their significance. Without a solid foundation of knowledge about EFM and the risks associated with repeated episodes of non-reassuring tracings, Alex and her husband don't realize they should be extremely concerned. They don't even know the appropriate questions to ask. They are young and unaccustomed to being proactive about their health care.

What they don't know can have serious repercussions for their family. Because they are uninformed, vital questions go unasked:

- Will this downward spiral continue?

- If it does, will our baby be able to bounce back?

- What is causing decelerations to keep reoccurring?

- What is causing the decreased variability (flattening out of the line indicating your baby's heart rate on the EFM tracing, instead of a saw tooth pattern)?

- What concerns does this non-reassuring pattern raise?

- What other actions can we take to stop the decelerations?

- Why is labor progressing so slowly?

- Why don't we just move to a C-section now, instead of continuing to expose our baby to the risk he may not be able to recover the next time his heart rate slows?

No one on the OB staff recognizes the seriousness of baby Nick's condition. No one concludes it is time to put a stop to this roller coaster ride of deterioration and improvement, although the baby's condition worsens and his recovery time lengthens with each episode. No one recognizes the dangers signaled by the length of time the induction is taking.

Baby Nick's heart rate drops again – this time, lower than before. He isn't getting an adequate amount of blood and oxygen through the placenta, and corrective measures clearly aren't working. Members of the OB staff finally recognize the baby is in severe distress and, with Alex's approval, an emergency delivery is ordered. Anesthesia, nursing and medical staff respond promptly, and a C-section is accomplished within twenty minutes.

A timely response to this emergency? Yes, but only after inappropriate obstetrical management allowed the emergency to develop. The failure to recognize and respond earlier to the downward spiral of Alex's baby has serious consequences. He suffers irreversible brain damage.

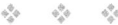

Looking on the brightest side possible, baby Nick suffered a less severe injury than do many babies in similar situations. While the brain damage he suffered manifested itself as cerebral palsy (typical with birth injuries of this nature), thankfully, Nick's cerebral palsy is mild.

Today, Nick is able to walk and run. His cognitive impairment places him at the borderline between low-normal and abnormal function levels. With the ongoing aid of caring, highly professional physical and occupational therapists, Nick's future is promising. With minimal assistance, he will be able to live a relatively normal life.

Nick is one of the luckier ones.

CHAPTER 10

What Went Wrong and Why

Introduction

Alex's story highlights complications that can occur with induction of labor, particularly if the use of induction agents causes contractions to become stronger or more frequent than a baby can tolerate. It also emphasizes that certain circumstances clearly indicate a baby is at greater-than-normal risk of being deprived of an adequate amount of oxygen during labor, whether or not labor has been induced. In baby Nick's case, those circumstances were repetitive, very low levels of amniotic fluid and decreased fetal movement. Each of these conditions is a warning sign the baby may not have sufficient stamina (sometimes characterized as *insufficient oxygen* or *insufficient fetal reserves*) to withstand even the rigors of natural, normal labor. Indeed, Alex's obstetrician decided to induce her labor three weeks before her due date specifically because he recognized the vulnerability associated with these conditions.

Further, by the time Nick was delivered, more than thirty-six hours had passed since the start of Alex's induction. Even more significantly, Alex was only four centimeters dilated, and Nick's head had not passed the -1 station.

Alex paid close attention to her baby's movement and did everything else correctly, as far as she knew, but it wasn't enough. Her obstetrical team failed to adequately appreciate and timely respond to EFM tracings signaling the need to cease labor induction and deliver baby Nick by C-section. This course of action should have been apparent, especially in light of Alex's history of low amniotic fluid, decreased fetal movement, and extremely slow labor progress. They also failed to adequately educate Alex about potential complications and risks to which her baby was exposed, and the warning signs they should have heeded far more quickly. With this information, Alex could have effectively advocated for better care for her baby.

Alex now fully understands she cannot rely on her birthing class or her obstetrical team to educate her about problems that can develop during labor and how to deal with them. She now knows it often takes an informed, proactive expectant mother to ensure a safe pregnancy and delivery.

Don't Be Prejudiced Against the Necessary C-Section

One thing Alex did correctly was not hesitate, even for a second, once the doctors told her a C-section was necessary. Remember how pleased she was at the beginning of her induction to hear a vaginal delivery was possible, despite decreased amniotic fluid and somewhat decreased fetal movement? She intuitively and smartly abandoned her preference as soon as she knew her baby was at risk. You should be prepared to do the same.

Classic First-Time Expectant Parents

Alex and her husband were the classic young couple experiencing the birth of their first child. Actually, their knowledge base about pregnancy, labor, and delivery was on a par with the overwhelming majority of pregnant women in this country, whether experiencing their first or fifth pregnancy.

Most women read some sort of publication about pregnancy. Unfortunately, they are all woefully inadequate and fail to convey the information necessary to help parents-to-be safeguard their babies' well-being.

Pregnancy is one part happiness and blissful expectation, one part uncertainty and worry. *Am I eating properly? Will my baby be healthy? Am I doing everything I can to ensure my baby's health and well-being?* Virtually everything published today is written in a touchy-feely manner designed to avoid upsetting the expectant mother.

But this approach doesn't give women the information they really need, much less answer the question, "Am I doing everything I can to ensure my baby's health and well-being?" Unfortunately, the answer is almost always, "No."

We believe you can handle the truth about potential complications, and we want to prepare you to deal with them. If having this knowledge causes you anguish, it pales in comparison to the heartache you would have if your baby suffered a birth injury that could have been avoided.

This chapter will focus on causes of decreased fetal movement, which may include the baby's sleep cycle; maternal conditions; use of prescription, over-the-counter, and illicit drugs; and the concept of fetal oxygen reserves. We will also discuss electronic fetal heart rate monitoring; appropriate interventions when faced with warning signs of fetal intolerance of labor; and the Friedman curve, which plots the normal time of labor against cervical dilation in both first-time and succeeding pregnancies.

Baby Nick's Decreased Fetal Oxygen Reserves Were Not Given Sufficient Concern

The well-being of mother and baby, and the appropriate course of action must always be weighed carefully, relative to the totality of the circumstances. This is the only way to reach a safe, appropriate conclusion.

Was Alex a candidate for induction of labor when she presented to the hospital? Yes, but those managing her care should have abandoned that trial well before baby Nick suffered any permanent injury from oxygen deprivation. That should have been obvious, based on the totality of the circumstances. What happened to this baby was entirely foreseeable, in light of a low level of amniotic fluid, decreased fetal movement, and the baby's inability to tolerate contractions well before they became more intense and were accompanied by maternal pushing (which significantly increases stress on the fetus). It should have been apparent this baby had limited oxygen reserves, to start with, and those reserves were becoming dangerously low as he was subjected to more and more stress. It was imperative to watch his EFM tracings particularly closely as Alex's labor progressed. In light of the circumstances, the threshold for abandoning labor and moving toward a surgical delivery should have been low.

Only Temporary Relief Was Achieved with Intrauterine Resuscitative Measures

The OB staff did a number of things right following the first episode of non-reassuring tracings. They decreased the dose of Pitocin they were administering, gave Alex oxygen and a bolus of fluids, repositioned her, and instituted the appropriate intrauterine resuscitative measures timely and appropriately. But these IURMs worked only temporarily.

The wisdom of allowing Alex's labor to resume after baby Nick's EFM became reassuring the second time can be debated, but there was no excuse for not discussing the situation openly and honestly with the parents at the time. Alex's obstetrician should have explained that labor would likely continue for at least six more hours, and the pushing phase during the last hour or two would become more intense, severely stressing the baby. Given the strain baby Nick had already undergone, the OB should have discouraged a vaginal delivery and strongly recommended a C-section. Alex would have consented to surgery, and a routine C-section would have been performed.

The wisdom of allowing this labor to resume – and worse yet, continuing to induce labor after he needed IURM for a third time – is not worthy of debate. Performing a C-section was the only reasonable course at that point.

If appropriate obstetrical management of Alex's induction of labor had been provided, baby Nick's oxygen would have remained at adequate levels. He would have been delivered safely, without any permanent injury.

Intrauterine Resuscitative Measures

As discussed earlier, intrauterine resuscitative measures are employed when the labor-and-delivery staff is concerned about some aspect of a fetal heart rate tracing. They consist of re-positioning the mother to either a left- or right-lateral position; administering oxygen through a facemask or nasal cannula; increasing IV fluids; and reducing, ceasing and/or reversing labor-inducing medications. If contractions don't slow after ceasing Pitocin or Cytotec, other medications can be given that act directly on the uterus to slow contractions. One of the final forms of IURM utilized is amnioinfusion, which entails placing a small tube into the uterine cavity and administering fluid to relieve pressure on the cord.

Any or all of these measures are frequently used during labor and delivery. It is important to understand why.

Often, IURM are used to resolve variable decelerations caused by compression of the umbilical cord. Changing the mother's position frequently accomplishes this goal, but amnioinfusion can be helpful if position change is unsuccessful. This is a reasonable approach, as long as the remainder of the tracing is reassuring. If the decelerations persist and become deeper, despite these maneuvers, reevaluation is necessary.

Once the baby's heart rate has recovered after IURM, the mother should find out exactly why resuscitative steps were taken. She must know the right question to ask: "Was there decreased variability in the baby's heart rate, late decelerations, or bradycardia?" (Remember, bradycardia is a heart rate below 110, commonly seen after an epidural is given.) Silence is not acceptable if the mother is to be proactive in protecting her baby's well-being.

An epidural can cause the mother's blood pressure to drop, frequently prompting a drop in the baby's heart rate. Intrauterine resuscitative measures will almost always correct this circumstance. However, if it is not corrected within five to ten minutes, the mother should insist on going to the operating room immediately. Once she is there, the baby's heart rate can be re-checked. If it has returned to normal, labor can be allowed to progress; if not, the baby should be delivered by emergency C-section.

CHAPTER 11

What Expectant Mothers Should Know About Fetal Movement, Fetal Oxygen Reserves, and Induction

More About the Significance of Electronic Fetal Monitoring

Fetal Movement

Lamaze® International advises women to let their "inner wisdom guide them through birth." We agree. Expectant mothers should call upon their instincts when it comes to their unborn baby's well-being, but not exclusively. Acquired knowledge about pregnancy and childbirth should guide them as well.

It is impossible to over-emphasize the importance of expectant mothers acting on their instincts. Although most concerns turn out to be nothing, mothers should never hesitate to raise them with their doctor because some concerns turn out to be very real. But there is something even more important than the mother's being proactive about speaking up, and that's making sure she is sufficiently informed to recognize appropriate concerns and know the right questions to ask.

During the third trimester, fetal movement becomes the most reliable marker of a baby's well-being. It is what brings the glow to the mother's face and leads her to wrap her arms around her belly. Fetal movement is a mother's first interaction with her baby, one that starts well before her child arrives. Just as babies speak to health care providers through fetal monitoring tracings, they speak to their mothers through movement within the womb.

Although mothers may feel the first flickering of movement as early as sixteen to eighteen weeks, it is not really until the third trimester – after twenty-eight weeks gestation – that movement becomes a reliable marker of a baby's well-being.

Normal Fetal Movement

On average, healthy babies move about thirty times an hour. Of course, not all these movements are perceived by the mother. Most moms, distracted by life's daily activities, don't give them much thought. When mothers are quiet, still and relaxed, they pay greater attention to their babies' activities.

It has been shown that a baby's most active time is usually during the late evening, typically from 9:00 p.m. to 1:00 a.m. This increased activity is thought to occur in response to decreased glucose levels in the mother's system.

Babies are also very sensitive to even slight changes in the amount of oxygen in their environments. Such changes have been shown to decrease babies' movements dramatically.

At twenty-eight weeks, the mother's obstetrical care provider should tell her it is time to start monitoring the baby's movements on a daily basis. Some will have her plot these movements on a fetal activity chart, but most will simply ask her to regularly count episodes of movement and immediately report any abnormalities.

Although different counting methods exist, the one most widely used – and the one we endorse – calls for the mother to be sure she feels her baby move at least ten times over a twelve-hour period. Fetal movement has been studied extensively, and this amount of activity has virtually a 100 percent correlation with a baby's intrauterine well-being.

Causes of Decreased Movement

Each baby has its own pattern of movement, and each mother comes to recognize her baby's pattern. Babies also have quiet times, mostly when sleeping or hungry for an extended period of time. That is why obstetricians always respond to phone calls about decreased fetal movement by instructing the mother to lie down on her side, eat and drink something sweet, and call back in thirty minutes to an hour if movement doesn't increase.

Other things can affect the ability of an expectant mother to perceive fetal movement. Mothers perceive their babies' movement most readily through the frontal part of the abdomen. Just as placing a pillow over one's stomach decreases the force and perception of a blow to that area, the natural cushions a mother's body develops decrease the perception of her baby's movements.

Certainly one of the most common factors in this decreased perception is the amount of fat a woman carries. The greater the amount of fatty tissue present, the less she will perceive fetal movement. Further, if the placenta is located toward the front of the mother's uterus, it also has a pillow-like effect, lessening the mother's ability to feel her baby move. Finally, as the volume of amniotic fluid surrounding the baby increases, the mother's perception of movement decreases.

Again, babies are very sensitive to even small changes in their oxygen supply. This is the final – and by far the most worrisome – cause of decreased fetal movement. As adults, we know that if oxygen is in short supply, cutting back on activity helps conserve it. Babies are no different; when their oxygen supply is insufficient, they also decrease their activity.

As you will recall, only a small amount of amniotic fluid surrounded Alex's baby, so if he was healthy and well-oxygenated, she should have had a heightened awareness of his movements. But because her fluid was low, the fact that she still perceived decreased fetal movement was a strong indicator of a problem with his well-being.

A baby gets its oxygen from its mother through the placenta and, eventually, the umbilical cord. Potential issues can arise at all or one of these sources. Some reverse themselves quickly, but others are chronic and demand close monitoring by ultrasound, EFM tracings, and the mother's perceptions of movement. Electronic fetal heart rate tracings taken after Alex entered the hospital revealed that, at least up to that point, baby Nick was tolerating his slightly decreased oxygen levels. As her labor progressed, those indications changed.

The bottom line: if you perceive your baby is less active than usual, you must call the doctor immediately, especially if you've been told your amniotic fluid level is low.

Conditions in Mom Affecting Baby's Movement

A number of conditions can potentially affect your baby's movement. The first has to do with what you ingest, which impacts what passes through the placenta and eventually reaches your baby.

Any sort of medication or substance that has a sedative effect on you will have the same effect on your baby. You probably know you should not use alcohol or illicit drugs such as marijuana or other depressive narcotics during pregnancy.

Common medications such as sleeping pills, antihistamines, cough medication and prescription pain medication may affect fetal movement, but shouldn't harm your baby if taken in accordance with appropriate directions. You should always discuss the effects of any medication, over-the-counter or prescribed, with your obstetrician before taking it. The best option is to take no medication whatsoever, but if you must do so, be sure you fully understand the potential consequences to your baby.

A number of chronic and acute medical problems in the mother may affect the amount of blood flow to the uterus and, therefore, the amount of oxygen delivered to her baby. Despite these medical issues, the baby often receives plenty of oxygen to assure its growth and well-being. These conditions and their potential effects should be well-known to your obstetrician and usually become more of a factor as pregnancy progresses. In addition to keeping an accurate fetal activity chart, the OB often arranges further testing to ensure the baby's health.

By far the most common of these worrisome conditions is hypertension (high blood pressure). It may be chronic, or it may occur acutely at some point during a pregnancy. There are many safe medications to treat hypertension during pregnancy.

The following applies to any and all medications taken during pregnancy: At a minimum, you should review the package insert that comes with the medication, paying particularly close attention to the warnings section. If you have Internet access, you should research the medication to determine whether credible questions have been raised about the drug's safety and discuss any concerns with your doctor prior to taking the medication.

Other illnesses that can potentially affect blood flow to the baby include diabetes with vascular changes; heart disease; lung disease; certain liver and gastrointestinal diseases; certain blood disorders, such as sickle cell or beta-thalassemia; and collagen vascular diseases.

If you have any of these illnesses, you should be followed by a perinatologist (an obstetrician with additional training, also referred to as a *high-risk obstetrician* or a *maternal-fetal medicine specialist*), rather than a general obstetrician.

Conditions in the Placenta

The placenta connects your blood supply to that of your baby. It also acts as a filter, allowing only certain things to cross and enter the baby's system. As previously noted, the placenta allows many medications to reach the baby, but it prevents others from doing so.

The placenta is an organ, just as the heart or lungs are organs. When it is healthy, the placenta grows and functions as it should, providing adequate oxygen and nutrients to your baby. But when the placenta is not healthy, the baby is at risk for an inadequate supply of oxygen.

The placenta grows by utilizing oxygen, hormones and nutrients supplied through maternal blood flow. Of these, blood flow is the most important factor. Many things affect the health of the placenta, most of which cannot be controlled. Some are produced by the mother's body, such as insulin and certain growth factors; others concern the maternal illnesses previously discussed; and still others involve where the placenta has implanted in the uterus.

The placenta's location is most commonly discovered during a routine second-trimester ultrasound. If a portion of the placenta covers the cervix (placenta previa) or is low-lying, the doctor should order a follow-up scan four to six weeks later to re-evaluate its position. Early in pregnancy, the uterus may only appear low because it is still relatively small. As pregnancy progresses and the uterus grows, follow-up scans usually demonstrate the placenta is actually in the middle portion of the uterus. Should the placenta remain low or over the cervix, the obstetrician should pay close attention to the baby's growth parameters.

Some women have uterine fibroid tumors. These tumors are almost always benign, solid, and mostly avascular (containing few or no blood vessels). Uterine fibroids can also be found outside the uterus, in the body or muscle of the uterus, or actually breaking through the muscle into the lining of the uterus, where the placenta implants. The closer the tumor is to the uterine lining, the more concerning it becomes. If a mother's placenta implants directly over a fibroid in this position, the blood supply is somewhat affected. Close monitoring, usually with ultrasound, is required.

How can you know whether your placenta is functioning properly? Decreased fetal activity is one sign, but the most common signal is inadequate fetal growth. The obstetrician measures the size of your uterus each time you visit to gauge your baby's growth. Should there be cause for concern, such as the growth rate being more than two weeks behind schedule, the doctor should perform an ultrasound to more accurately assess your baby's size. If the placenta is found to be abnormally small, the ultrasound should be repeated every two or three weeks to ensure continued growth. Should any one of these follow-up exams show no growth, an immediate delivery is indicated.

The Umbilical Cord

The umbilical cord floats freely in the amniotic cavity, and is attached to the placenta at one end and the baby at the other. The blood vessels in the cord carry oxygen and nutrients to the baby and waste products away from the baby. Obviously, compression of the cord may potentially decrease the baby's oxygen supply and activity level.

Compression can occur in several ways. It is very common for babies to become entangled in the umbilical cord, causing it to wrap around their neck, arm or leg. Babies usually untangle themselves, with no consequences. Nearly 20 percent of babies are born with the umbilical cord around their necks. (This is called a *nuchal cord*.) However, there are times when compression of the umbilical cord affects blood flow to the baby, causing decreased activity.

Blood flow to your baby can also be affected by where the cord inserts into the placenta. The closer the point of insertion is to the edge of the placenta (eccentric location), the greater the risk of an adverse effect on blood flow. The location of the umbilical cord is one of the things routinely checked during the second-trimester ultrasound. Even if told the ultrasound is entirely normal, you should always inquire about the location of the placenta and umbilical cord.

Closing Comments on Fetal Activity

Keeping track of fetal movement is of paramount importance. You should monitor it daily and call your doctor sooner, not later, if you have any concerns about your baby's activity.

Alex's reporting decreased movement in her baby sparked closer monitoring and prompted her doctor to deliver baby Nick three weeks early. Had she not reported this when she did, it's highly possible her baby would not have survived until the natural onset of labor. Unfortunately, the nurses and physicians attending Alex at the hospital did not heed the worrisome signs on the fetal monitor strips. These tracings clearly revealed baby Nick had not been getting adequate oxygen, a circumstance he was no longer able to withstand.

Electronic Fetal Monitoring

Alex's story highlights complications that can occur with the induction of labor, particularly if the use of induction agents causes contractions to become too strong or too frequent. It further highlights your baby's vulnerability to being deprived of adequate oxygen during labor – whether or not labor is induced – when amniotic fluid is very low and fetal movement is diminished. Under such circumstances, your baby may not have sufficient stamina or oxygen reserves to withstand even the rigors of natural, normal labor.

This expectant mother (FIG. 2) is undergoing external EFM. The two devices necessary to perform this monitoring are attached to the mother's abdomen by elastic bands. The transducer, attached to the lower band, uses ultrasound to keep track of the fetal heart rate. Ultrasonic waves from the transducer pass through the mother's abdomen and are reflected back to the device by the baby's heart. The tocodynamometer (toco), attached to the upper band, detects uterine contractions. When the uterine muscle contracts, the toco records it from beginning to end. The box-like piece of equipment on the table

(FIG. 2)

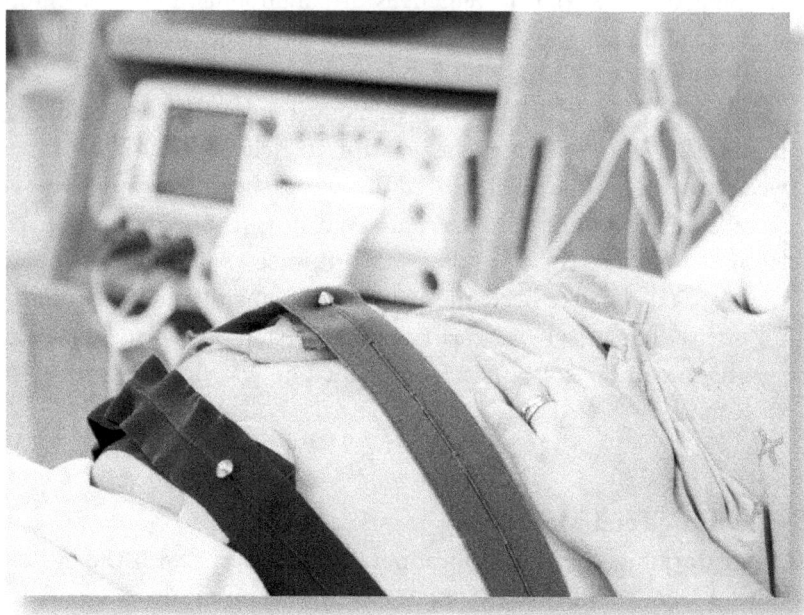

next to the bed receives signals from both devices and prints paper strips graphing the results. Both graphs appear on a single piece of paper.

As stated earlier, babies communicate with the outside world through electronic fetal monitor tracings. An entire chapter of this book is devoted to teaching the basics of EFM. You should take the time to study it carefully, as it may be the most important thing you do to ensure your baby's safety during labor and delivery.

At the very minimum, you should know how to recognize your baby's baseline heart rate on an EFM tracing, as well as the difference between good variability (a saw tooth pattern) versus decreased or absent variability (almost a straight line). You should immediately question a decrease in your baby's baseline heart rate of ten or more beats per minute. You should also question decreased or absent variability for more than twenty to thirty minutes.

You should not accept the answer, "Don't worry, it's totally normal." Insist on an explanation of the cause of the decrease and why it is normal. Remember, if you are placed on your side or given oxygen, this means something in your baby's tracing is definitely not normal, and you should demand more information. If Pitocin is being administered, make sure it is stopped.

If these intrauterine resuscitative measures are performed, it is very important to have a conversation with your doctor about the estimated time until delivery. If delivery is anticipated soon, and the baby's heart rate has responded, continuing labor is probably fine. On the other hand, if the anticipated delivery is remote, and the labor induction is secondary to low amniotic fluid or a small or growth-restricted baby, a C-section should be seriously considered.

CHAPTER 12

Questions to Ask and Subjects to Review with Your Obstetrician

Pregnancy is mostly a time of happiness and bonding, not only between you and your baby as you feel it growing inside you, but also between you and loved ones as you joyously plan for your baby's arrival. But inevitably, mothers experience times of concern. These concerns range from simple issues, like whether the hospital will allow videotaping of the delivery, to much more serious ones, such as decreases in your baby's movements. It is critically important to have an obstetrician who is willing address all concerns about your baby's well-being.

Many of these worries arise unexpectedly and can wait until your next regularly scheduled appointment. Just be sure to write them down, so you don't forget them. For more pressing concerns, you must ensure the communication lines are open, day and night, between you and your doctor.

Fetal Movement

- One of the expectant mother's most important concerns is the perception of a change in her baby's activity level. Early in the third trimester, have a detailed discussion with your doctor about what constitutes a normal activity level and when you should be concerned.

- What should you do if you perceive a decrease in your baby's movement? This is a very important conversation. Your doctor's response should always be to call sooner, not later.

- Be sure you are clear on how to reach your obstetrician all the time, especially after office hours, and keep all necessary numbers with you at all times.

- How long after you call should you expect a response? Even after office hours, you should never have to wait more than fifteen minutes after a call involving an urgent concern.

- What should you do if you can't reach your obstetrician doctor? Occasionally, your doctor may be involved in another delivery or surgery, and unable to return your call in a timely manner. Be sure you have a backup number for urgent questions. Many times, this will be the direct number to the hospital's labor-and-delivery department.

- If you are having an ultrasound during the third trimester, be sure to ask the technician or doctor performing the exam to check for a nuchal cord (umbilical cord around your baby's neck). As stated earlier, this is a fairly common occurrence. If this condition exists, no extra testing is necessary, but you should be aware any sign of decreased fetal movement must be immediately addressed with electronic fetal monitoring or ultrasound.

- What if decreased fetal movement is a recurring concern? Whether the first or fifth occurrence, unresolved decreased movement always requires fetal monitoring. If it occurs more than once, insist on an ultrasound, as well.

Decreased Amniotic Fluid

- One of the early signs of decreased amniotic fluid is a discrepancy between your dates and uterine measurement (fundal height). Starting at about twenty-four weeks, always ensure your fundal height is measured, and ask for the results. In centimeters, this measurement should be about equal to your current week of pregnancy. A one- to two-centimeter difference is normal, but any larger disparity or a recurrent lag of two centimeters should be investigated with an ultrasound. If a disparity is found, ask your doctor what is causing it.

- Is the underlying cause treatable? At minimum, decreased amniotic fluid requires immediate bed rest and follow-up scans.

- What testing should be done? A variety of tests may be performed to ensure your baby's well-being, such as a non-stress test (NST), a biophysical profile (BPP), and a contraction stress test (CST), each of which is defined in the Glossary of Obstetrical Terms. Your most important concern is being sure these tests are conducted at least on a weekly basis.

- Is a vaginal delivery safe? Be sure your obstetrician understands you wish an immediate C-section to be performed if your baby isn't tolerating labor and that very serious problem cannot be timely and reliably corrected.

Electronic Fetal Monitoring

- When you are in labor and electronic fetal monitoring is being conducted, review your baby's tracing and your understanding of EFM with your doctor or nurse. Be sure you have an understanding of the basics, such as baseline, variability, contraction pattern, accelerations, and decelerations.

- If intrauterine resuscitative measures are performed, be sure you understand why, and insist on knowing the results.

- Be sure open lines of communication exist among you, the nurse and your provider. Don't assume an attitude of knowing as much about monitoring as they do; you don't. By the same token, be sure they know you do understand it somewhat, you learned this for your baby's safety, and you want any concerns to be addressed openly, fully and hospitably.

- Again, stress that your baby's safety is your number-one concern. You want a C-section to be performed sooner, rather than later, in the face of worrisome tracings.

PART V

Prenatal Testing and Care: How to Earn an "A"

CHAPTER 13

Sara's Story

(As Told from the Perspective of Dr. Giles H. Manley)
Some patients are simply unforgettable. Sara is one of them. Is she so memorable because of the roller coaster ride of highs and lows we shared during her prenatal care? Or is it because I am proud of myself for making a difficult diagnosis that easily could have gone unnoticed and resulted in catastrophe? Most likely, it is a combination of the two.

A young couple sits in my office for the first time, obviously a bit nervous. Sara and her husband, Jim, are holding hands. They are also holding two pages of questions they want me to answer.

A little light banter about their lives, jobs and family eases their tension. I assure them all questions will be addressed and ask them to let me take the lead.

Sara and Jim have been married for five years. Financially and emotionally, they are ready for children. It's obvious they are planners who take nothing for granted. Sara is about seven weeks along with their first baby. They want to have two children.

As they sit before me, the young couple can barely contain their excitement. Jim tells me their parents are all equally thrilled, as this will be the first grandchild for both Sara's parents and his own. He explains that he and his wife are both only children, and that is why they feel so strongly about having a second child – so each of the siblings will have a companion, friend, and confident to share all that life brings their way.

By the end of the visit, we have covered all Jim's and Sara's questions. They are far more relaxed and seem comfortable with me as their obstetrician. Before they leave, I instruct Sara to get various types of lab work done, including a compete blood count (CBC), and return for a follow-up exam in five weeks.

On the next visit, Sara returns alone, as Jim is traveling on business. Once again, she has a list of questions – fortunately, only one page this time. During Sara's examination, we hear her baby's heartbeat for the first time. Initially, she smiles from ear to ear, but her smile soon disappears, as she realizes Jim isn't here to share this milestone. At my suggestion, she phones her husband, and her unbridled joy returns as Jim listens remotely to the rhythmic sounds of the baby's heart.

Afterward, we return to my office to go over Sara's lab results, which reveal she is slightly anemic. This is not particularly worrisome; many women are anemic due to blood loss secondary to their menstrual cycles, combined with not enough iron intake. However, the lab report also shows Sara's blood cells are slightly smaller than normal, a finding not explained by iron-deficient anemia. Probing Sara's family history in greater depth reveals new information: she is of Mediterranean descent. For this reason, we need to run another blood test to determine whether she is a carrier of a certain gene that can cause a serious genetic disease called *beta-thalassemia*, which is similar to sickle-cell anemia. This gene is more common in persons of Mediterranean or Asian ancestry than in other segments of the population. A carrier is a person who has only one of two genes required for a disease to develop. Carriers often are unaware they have the gene, as they typically have no symptoms associated with it.

I explain to Sara that even a positive test result shouldn't be problematic, as both parents must be carriers of the gene for their baby to be at risk for any genetic disorder. Given her husband's physical characteristics, it's extremely unlikely he would be a carrier, too. Sara is comforted, but still leaves feeling a bit apprehensive.

The results of Sara's second set of blood work confirm she is, indeed, a carrier for beta-thalassemia. My nurse calls to ask Sara and Jim to come in at the end of my day's schedule. This sort of information should not be delivered by phone. Two hours later, they sit before me, holding hands, anticipating bad news.

Although I reassure them, something in Jim's medical history troubles me. He reported that the Red Cross once turned him down as a blood donor. Out of an abundance of caution, I send him for testing as well. Surprisingly, the lab reports he also is a carrier.

Sara and Jim are obviously shaken. And indeed, this news is difficult to hear. More than likely, Sara's and Jim's baby is fine, but there is a 25 percent chance the child has beta-thalassemia. Children with the severe form of the disease require a lifetime of frequent transfusions and a variety of other procedures to help them remain as healthy as possible; however, many do not reach age forty.

Sara and Jim listen carefully as I explain the next steps. We can immediately perform an amniocentesis for genetic testing of the baby. The test involves inserting a long needle through the abdomen and uterus into the amniotic sac and withdrawing fluid. But it carries risks. Depending on operator experience, one in 200-1,600 patients miscarry. This range is so large because of a wide variance in operating experience. Some doctors perform as few as one or two procedures a year, while others perform hundreds each year. Expectant mothers should search out and opt for experienced operators, whenever possible.

Sara and Jim listen quietly. They fully comprehend that if tests confirm their baby has beta-thalassemia, there is ample time to terminate the pregnancy, should they elect to do so. "These decisions can be difficult," I begin to say, but before I can complete the thought, almost in unison, Jim and Sara declare, "That's not for us. It's not in our DNA." With abortion off the table, the only question remaining is whether they want to conduct the testing anyway, so they will know what to expect when the baby is born.

It is Friday, and Jim and Sara decide to take the weekend to reflect on whether she should undergo the amniocentesis. Although the risks of a miscarriage are small, they must answer this question: *Knowing they won't terminate the pregnancy, regardless of the test results, could they live with themselves if Sara were to miscarry a healthy baby as a result of the test?*

Sara and Jim return to my office on Monday. They both look exhausted. Coming to grips with their situation and agonizing over whether to undergo the test clearly has exacted a toll. Ultimately, they have decided they need to know. They hope the test will be safe and produce negative results, giving them peace of mind concerning their baby's well-being.

On Wednesday, Sara undergoes the amniocentesis without incident, much to everyone's relief. When the lab results come back, the news couldn't be better. Jim's and Sara's baby does not have beta-thalassemia, but is only a carrier. They are elated.

I will never forget their tears of relief, their gratitude, and the absolute joy Sara and Jim displayed in my office that day. A few months later, Sara delivered a bouncing, healthy little boy, James Jr.

I still get a Christmas card from Sara and Jim every year. Mom, dad and son are all doing well. Although they had hoped to have a second baby, Sara and Jim decided they could not go through this experience again or be responsible for potentially bringing a child into the world, only to experience the suffering that goes along with beta-thalassemia. Sara's husband had a vasectomy a year after her delivery.

CHAPTER 14

What Went Right and Why

Sara and Jim were diligent in researching and selecting a hospital. Although they lived within five minutes of a facility with an obstetrical department, they decided to consider other factors, as well. They meticulously investigated the hospital closest to their home, along with five others within an hour's drive. They looked at things such as anesthesia coverage, nursery capabilities, number of deliveries performed, and obstetrical in-house coverage. In the end, they selected the hospital where I practiced.

Sara and Jim were equally diligent in choosing their obstetrician. They called a number of practices to get a feel for the right fit. Their decision was influenced even by such things as how they were greeted and treated by staff during their initial phone calls. When we first met, I was attentive, answered all their questions, did not rush through the visit, and reassured them they would always be able to reach me easily. As was my habit with all my obstetrical and surgical patients, I gave them my cell phone number. I assured them if they had to go to the hospital in case of emergency, they might be seen by another doctor, but I would make sure their care was coordinated expediently and appropriately. Over twenty years of practice, my patients have rarely abused this privilege.

I was thorough in my observations about the results of Sara's bloodwork and followed through on a nagging hunch. Although

Sara had certain very subtle Mediterranean characteristics, neither she nor her blonde-haired husband identified themselves as such. Although in their initial visit, I didn't ask either of them about their heritage – particularly not about Jim's, given his appearance – the results of Sara's CBC raised my suspicion. The results didn't reflect an iron deficiency, which would have explained her mild anemia, but certain other blood factors were slightly abnormal. When Sara returned for her next visit, I did question her about her ancestry, and she confirmed her grandparents were from Italy. On further testing, her bloodwork showed she was a carrier of one gene for beta-thalassemia.

I felt it was highly unlikely Jim was also a carrier, but if he was, the baby would be at significant risk for this life-altering disease. So I followed through and called the young parents in for a visit. Questions about Jim's ancestry did not reveal a Mediterranean or Eastern European background; however, with a little more probing, he revealed a history of not being a viable blood donor due to mild anemia – another red flag. I arranged to have Jim's blood tested. Sure enough, the results showed he was also a carrier of the gene for beta-thalassemia. This meant Sara's and Jim's child had a one in four chance of having the disease.

Thankfully, the amniocentesis we performed showed Jim's and Sara's baby was only a carrier, as were his parents. They were tremendously relieved and went on to have a healthy delivery.

This story might easily have had a very different outcome. Had Jim and Sara not been so conscientious in choosing a hospital and an OB, the issue of ancestry might have gone unnoticed in examining the results of Sara's blood work. Had I not been diligent in my observations and in taking their medical histories, as well as in checking the blood characteristics for anemia type (something many physicians don't do), their carrier status might have only been learned after the birth of a very sick baby.

Selecting a Physician and Hospital

When selecting an obstetrician, be sure to ask how often they are on duty in the hospital and who covers for them when they are not available. Ask questions about how easily they can be reached, how many babies they have delivered, who will see you for most of your visits, and any other questions that help you feel comfortable with the doctor.

Although you may want to meet every doctor who might possibly deliver your baby, this is not a good idea. It is much safer to see one doctor for most of your visits, as this will minimize the chance of important lab work or testing going unnoticed.

Do careful online research about your primary OB, as well as the backup physician. You can find out from your state medical board whether any lawsuits are pending against a doctor. If either your doctor or the backup physician is the subject of three or more legal actions, you should thoroughly investigate the circumstances.

If possible, choose a hospital with a round-the-clock, in-house anesthesia team. If you use a midwife, make sure the birth will take place in a hospital, not a birthing center, so you will have immediate access to a fully equipped and staffed operating room in case an emergency C-section is necessary.

If at all possible, choose a hospital that has a neonatal intensive care unit (NICU). A well-trained NICU staff in a fully equipped NICU suite can make a critical difference in your baby's outcome if a serious complication develops. These medical professionals have specialized training and experience, and are in the best position to diagnose a problem and provide the treatment your baby needs immediately. Avoiding the delay associated with having to transfer your baby to a facility with a neonatal intensive care unit can minimize or avoid altogether permanent injury to your newborn.

CHAPTER 15

What Expectant Mothers Should Know

Prenatal Tests

An ultrasound should be conducted during the first obstetrical visit to determine the due date. It should be repeated at eighteen to twenty weeks, when the fetal anatomy becomes clear enough to see anomalies.

Your obstetrician will order a routine urinalysis, cultures, and blood work on your first visit or shortly afterward. These tests check for anemia; sexually transmitted diseases, such as gonorrhea, syphilis, chlamydia and HIV; rubella (to check your immunity to measles); your blood type; and other conditions that might affect you or your baby. This routine lab work does not test for every possible condition, so if there is anything in your partner's or your history (such as not being allowed to donate blood) that is even slightly out of the ordinary, be sure to tell your doctor about it on your first visit.

If there is any possibility at all you could have been exposed to herpes at some time in your life, request a blood test for this condition. In fact, we recommend all pregnant women be tested for herpes.

If you are of Eastern European, Mediterranean, Asian or African descent, you should alert your obstetrician so you can be screened to determine if you are a carrier for certain genetic conditions. For example, women of African descent should be screened for sickle-cell disease. If you are a carrier for a genetic condition, the father should immediately undergo genetic testing for the same condition. If he is also a carrier, your baby is at risk for being a carrier or even inheriting the disorder.

As you age, the number of healthy eggs in your ovaries decreases, and the number of eggs with chromosomal abnormalities increases. Down syndrome is an example of a condition associated with a chromosomal defect. If you become pregnant at age 33 or older, the risk of your fetus' having a damaged chromosome is high enough to warrant considering fetal testing.

At about sixteen weeks into your pregnancy, you will be offered a blood test to screen for genetic abnormalities. Be aware these blood tests may produce false-positive results. You should also be aware assessing the presence of genetic defects in a fetus requires invasive testing that could potentially cause a miscarriage.

If you are pregnant or ready to attempt to become pregnant, and there is reason to be concerned about genetic issues associated with pregnancy, both you and your partner should be offered genetic counseling. Effective counseling should enable you and your partner to make informed decisions with respect to becoming pregnant, testing, and possibly terminating the pregnancy in the event fetal testing results are unfavorable.

Your weight may trigger the need to undergo certain prenatal screening. If you weigh more than 200 pounds, be sure you are screened for diabetes in both the first and second trimesters. First-trimester screening is conducted to ascertain if you have undiagnosed diabetes. Second-trimester screening determines whether you have developed pregnancy-related diabetes (gestational diabetes) due to hormonal changes that occur during this time period.

First and Second Trimester

You should expect to see your doctor every four to six weeks until you are twenty-eight weeks pregnant. At that point, the frequency of your visits should increase to every three weeks, then every two weeks, and finally, once a week for the last three weeks before delivery.

Fetal movement should begin at fifteen to eighteen weeks. As mentioned above, at twenty-four to twenty-eight weeks, all expectant mothers should be tested for diabetes because the placenta produces a substance that can affect how glucose is metabolized.

There are four blood types – O, A, B, and AB. Just as a magnet has a positive and negative pole, each of the blood types is either positive or negative. For instance, you can be O-negative or O-positive, but not both. The positives and negatives don't mix; if you have negative blood and positive blood is introduced into your system, your body will destroy those positive blood cells.

During pregnancy, some of your baby's blood cells will enter your system, especially in the third trimester and during delivery. If they are not destroyed quickly, your body will eventually destroy them, and then form antibodies that can potentially harm future pregnancies. RhoGAM is an injection that lasts twelve weeks, and will destroy any positive cells in your body before you have time to form potentially harmful antibodies.

Know your blood type. If you are Rh-negative, have the baby's father tested. If he is Rh-positive, RhoGAM should be injected at twenty-eight weeks and re-injected after delivery if your baby is also Rh positive. Failure to receive the second injection could risk future pregnancies, so keep demanding it until you get it. Also, should you have any bleeding episodes at any time in your pregnancy, it is important to remind your OB immediately that you are Rh-negative.

Expectant mothers are routinely tested at thirty-two to thirty-six weeks for group B strep bacteria, which is the primary cause of meningitis in newborns. If you test positive, you won't treated for this bacteria until you are in labor. In this case, be sure to immediately ask for treatment when you are admitted to the hospital. If necessary, don't hesitate to repeatedly inform the OB staff that you tested positive. You should be given IV antibiotics without delay.

Abnormal pain, any vaginal bleeding, unusual pressure or abnormal discharge at any time during pregnancy should always be brought to the attention of your doctor immediately. Discharge with odor can be bacterial vaginitis, which can lead to premature labor if left untreated. Urinary tract infections are common and must be treated right away, as pregnancy speeds this infection to the kidneys.

There are several other important matters to consider. Sexual intercourse is safe unless your doctor tells you otherwise. Spotting afterward may occur occasionally and is almost always harmless, but if it persists for longer than a few days or gets heavier, notify your doctor immediately. Take your prenatal vitamins. If you go out of town, take a copy of your chart (only the history and physical pages, along with the visit flow sheet and lab summary sheet) in case of complications. Take a tour of the hospital sooner rather than later. Finally, write down questions and concerns as you think of them; otherwise, you may forget them by the time you see your obstetrician.

The Third Trimester
If you notice any decrease in your baby's activity during the last three months of pregnancy, contact your doctor immediately. Your may be advised to eat something sweet and lie on your left side, which usually causes the baby's movement to quickly return to normal. If it doesn't, call back immediately and insist on going to the hospital and being connected to a fetal heart monitor. Do not feel guilty about bothering your doctor after hours or insisting on hospital admission for monitoring. Any change in your baby's activity late in pregnancy should be of great concern. This is no time to be shy or intimidated.

If you develop medical issues during the third trimester that warrant fetal monitoring, and you are told you may need to be induced because the test results are worrisome or non-reassuring, demand a C-section. Worrisome fetal testing usually means your baby is stressed and not receiving enough oxygen. In such a case, your baby's reserves or ability to withstand further stressors, such as uterine contractions, may be compromised. Although your baby may well be able to withstand labor, is it really worth finding out? Do not risk the health of your unborn child over a misplaced belief that one form of delivery is better than another.

The third trimester is also the time to attend a class to learn about the labor-and-delivery process. These classes may be offered at your hospital or elsewhere in the community. Birthing classes can be memorable and empowering, and we recommend all first-time mothers and their partners seriously consider taking them. Lamaze® International and similar birthing classes help expectant parents understand the birthing process, teach valuable techniques for easing the pain of labor and delivery, and help fathers or partners take an active role in pregnancy and delivery. However, as we explained previously, educating parents-to-be about potentially serious obstetrical complications is not the focus of their curriculum.

Remember, pregnancy should be a wonderful time in your life. We suggest you encourage your partner to accompany you to as many doctor visits as possible. It will make your partner feel more a part of this wonderful process and help with bonding, once the baby arrives. If your partner doesn't wish to attend, or if you have no partner, ask a friend or family member to accompany you. For your emotional health, it is important to share this experience with someone close to you.

CHAPTER 16

Questions to Ask Your Obstetrician

Here's a list of important questions to ask before choosing an obstetrician and hospital:

- How can I reach the doctor when the office is closed?

- What other doctors cover for my obstetrician, and how experienced are they?

- May I meet these backup doctors?

- At what hospital does my obstetrician deliver? If my OB delivers babies at more than one hospital, what happens if he or she is busy in a different hospital when I go into labor?

- Does the hospital have a NICU, and if so, what is the earliest gestational age it can handle? (Some NICUs only accept babies over twenty-eight weeks of gestational age.)

- Does the hospital have a perinatologist (high-risk obstetrician) on staff? If not, what happens if I need a consult?

- Is an anesthesiologist on duty at the hospital twenty-four hours a day, seven days a week? If not, what happens if I require anesthesia at a time when no anesthesiologist is on duty?

- Do I have your assurance I will be given the results of any lab, ultrasound or other testing performed on me or my baby?

- How many people are allowed in the delivery room? How many are allowed in the operating room?

PART VI

Is Using a Midwife a Mistake?

Prolonged Rupture of Membranes
Poses a Risk of Infection

CHAPTER 17

Marjeta's Story

Early on the morning of December 1, Marjeta is in the midst of a deep, restful slumber when she is awakened by a warm, wet sensation. Groggy and confused, she climbs out of bed to find her nightgown and sheets soaked. She reaches for the lamp and nudges her husband. "Wake up. The baby is coming."

Within minutes, Marjeta realizes something is strange. Her water has broken, but she has had no contractions. *Contractions are supposed to come first. Then the water.* An hour passes with no other indication of labor. Marjeta calls the birthing center to report the spontaneous rupture of her amniotic membranes. The nurse midwife with whom she speaks tells her to come in the next morning.

Marjeta is thirty-six weeks into her second pregnancy. She has already named her little girl Jana, meaning "God's gracious gift, harvest of fruit." She wanted a natural birth with her first child, but circumstances made it necessary to deliver by C-section. So when Marjeta learned she was pregnant a second time, she again hoped for a natural delivery.

Early in her pregnancy, Marjeta consulted with the staff at a birthing center near her home. She authorized the nurse midwife to obtain her hospital records to clarify why a C-section had been necessary with her first child and determine whether it would be safe to attempt a natural birth with Jana. Marjeta also questioned the midwife about the safety of a vaginal birth following a C-section (VBAC).

Months later, the midwife assured Marjeta the records contained nothing to indicate any problem with attempting a vaginal delivery and said it appeared the C-section she underwent had not been absolutely necessary. She told Marjeta many obstetricians are impatient about letting nature take its course and rush to perform a C-section when a woman's labor progresses slowly.

Now, as she arrives at the birthing center early on the morning of December first, Marjeta is concerned she may have to undergo another C-section. *My water broke hours ago, so why hasn't my labor begun?*

The midwife confirms the amniotic membranes have ruptured and conducts a non-stress test verifying the baby's well-being. She tells Marjeta spontaneous rupture is common and nothing to worry about. "Come back tomorrow," she says.

But Marjeta is concerned about Jana's safety. She persists with the discussion, asking about the risks of waiting, as opposed to inducing labor now by administering Pitocin. The midwife assures her there is no reason for concern and insists it is usually better to allow labor to begin on its own.

On December 2, Marjeta returns to the birthing center, where the same exam is repeated, with the same results. The midwife again instructs her to return the next day or when contractions begin, whichever comes first.

Marjeta does as she is told, but cannot shake her concern. Although she has dreamed of a natural birth, she cannot jeopardize her baby girl's safety. On December 3, the young mother returns to the birthing center, her mind made up: "If my labor doesn't start tonight," she tells the midwife, "I want to have a C-section tomorrow."

That evening, she feels a little warm and detects some mild tenderness in her abdomen. Soon afterward, Marjeta goes into labor. She arrives at the birthing center at 9:45 p.m. on December 3. At this point, it has been two full days since her amniotic membranes ruptured.

The midwife connects her to the external fetal monitor for a short time and takes her vital signs. Marjeta hears Jana's heartbeat and sees its tracings on the EFM printout. Relief washes over her, but it is short-lived. Marjeta notices Jana's heart rate is higher than usual, fluctuating between 160 and 170 beats per minute, and questions the midwife.

Again, the midwife tells her there is no reason for concern, and even says the EFM tracing is very reassuring. Marjeta has a low-grade temperature, which could be contributing to Jana's slightly elevated heart rate. She performs a vinegar douche, explaining it will help prevent infection.

The midwife's manner and assurances are very calming, and Marjeta finally begins to relax. *After all, she has been doing this for over twenty years. She has delivered hundreds of babies. She knows what she's talking about.*

Over the next several hours, Marjeta's contractions become stronger and much more frequent. Periodically, the midwife checks Jana's heart with a stethoscope-like device called a *Doptone*. Although comforted each time she hears it, Marjeta still has a nagging concern. *Jana's heartbeat seems so fast.*

Shortly after 1:00 a.m., Marjeta's temperature rises to 101 degrees Fahrenheit. About this time, the midwife tells her it is time to push. *The midwife is calm, so surely things are fine.*

After receiving instructions about the proper way to push, Marjeta starts bearing down with all her might. The midwife encourages her and checks Jana's heartbeat every few minutes. She has explained to Marjeta that pushing may put more stress on the baby, so more frequent monitoring is necessary.

Within about fifteen minutes, Jana's heart rate slows considerably. The midwife instructs Marjeta to stop pushing for a bit. She repositions Marjeta in the bed, moving her onto her right side. She then begins administering fluids intravenously and applies a nasal cannula to give Marjeta supplemental oxygen. She re-checks Jana's heart rate, which has returned to its previous fast pace. Marjeta thinks she detects a shadow of concern on the midwife's face.

Following orders, Marjeta again begins to push. But within a few minutes, the electronic fetal monitor shows Jana's heart rate has slowed again – this time, to seventy – and it doesn't rebound when Marjeta stops pushing.

The midwife lacks the knowledge, training and ability to do anything more. Her only recourse is to dial 911.

After what seems an eternity, Marjeta is finally transported by ambulance to a nearby hospital. The midwife has called ahead, and the doctors and nurses are awaiting her arrival. They immediately perform an ultrasound and find Jana is fighting for her life, but just barely hanging on. Her heart rate is now in the range of twenty to forty beats per minute.

Marjeta is rushed into the operating room, given general anesthesia, and Jana is born within a few minutes. The baby is limp, blue, and not breathing. She has no heartbeat. For twenty-five minutes, the doctors work tirelessly to revive her. At one point, a faint heartbeat returns, but only for a few fleeting minutes.

After nearly a half-hour of extraordinary efforts to save Jana, they call an end to the code. A few hours later, in the recovery room, Marjeta says a permanent goodbye to her baby girl.

The autopsy report states Jana's cause of death as asphyxia caused by an overwhelming infection, group B sepsis.

CHAPTER 18

What Went Wrong and Why

Introduction

For some women, delivering naturally is not even a consideration. In fact, many mothers now elect to deliver by C-section. They make this choice for a variety of reasons, including convenience, avoiding labor, and concerns about incontinence, just to mention a few.

However, most woman feel just as Marjeta did. Whether culturally motivated or instinctive, their preference for a vaginal birth is strong, and many want the birth to be as natural and drug-free as possible. Many believe natural childbirth is best achieved with a midwife.

Marjeta's midwife confirmed what she had always suspected – that her first C-section had not been necessary. She had been raised to believe a natural delivery was a badge of honor – the epitome of womanhood. She spoke at length with her midwife, who answered all her questions and met all her concerns with such reassurance, empathy, and comfort that she felt entirely confident planning to deliver at the birthing center. Marjeta loved the peaceful décor and the freedom of not being strapped to a bed. And she was comforted by knowing a hospital and a doctor were nearby.

Unfortunately, Marjeta was lulled into a false sense of security. Choosing to use a midwife was safe. Choosing to deliver outside a hospital was not.

We firmly believe it is never acceptable to plan to give birth anywhere except in a hospital. As in Marjeta's case, when an emergency arises, every minute is precious to your baby's health and survival. In the twenty-five minutes it took to get Marjeta to the hospital, Jana suffered fatal brain damage, exacerbated by her concurrent bacterial infection with group B streptococcus.

This chapter will cover midwifery and birthing centers. We will explore the strong advantages of choosing a midwife for certain patients, as well as some of the potential downsides. Every midwife must be backed up by an obstetrician. In fact, Marjeta's midwife did have an obstetrical backup, but she waited too long to enlist the OB's help. In the following pages, we will discuss situations in which women using a midwife must insist on an obstetrical consult. Finally, we will cover infection and premature rupture of membranes – when it is acceptable to await the natural onset of labor and when it is not.

Birthing Centers

Babies are sensitive to certain environments, so we understand your desire to have your baby experience labor and delivery in as serene a setting as possible. For exactly this reason, most U.S. hospitals have upgraded from the sterile labor rooms of old to much more comfortable, spacious and inviting birthing suites.

Regardless, some women still identify hospitals with stress and discomfort, and find a birthing center far more appealing. A birthing center provides a relaxing setting, undisturbed by nurses, intercoms, and often-unfamiliar health professionals coming into the labor suite. Such an atmosphere is private and soothing for both mother and baby.

We fully admit it: In most cases, giving birth in a birthing center is a happy, fulfilling experience with a positive outcome. But our job is to educate. Once we have done that, the rest is up to you.

We have no issues with birthing centers located inside hospitals. Our concerns are focused on free-standing birthing centers. Even a birthing center located on a hospital's grounds, but outside the main facility, is still too risky.

If a true emergency arises, minutes – sometimes even seconds – are critical to your baby's health and survival. Even when a center is located on a hospital campus, at least twenty minutes can be lost by the time you are moved from the birthing center to the operating room. For Marjeta's baby, Jana, this twenty-five-minute transfer was fatal.

Think about it: you are in a free-standing center, in the midst of labor. You are not at your agile best. An emergency call is made, and help arrives within a few minutes, if you are lucky. The emergency responders must bring a stretcher into the building, quickly assess the situation, transfer you to the stretcher, move you out of the building and into the ambulance, drive the short distance to the hospital, transfer you to a hospital stretcher, and rush you to the emergency suite. Once there, doctors and nurses quickly re-assess your condition and that of your baby, and you are finally transported to the operating room, where you are transferred to the operating table.

If you are extraordinarily lucky, this is all accomplished within twenty minutes, but thirty to forty minutes is the norm. When your baby is deprived of oxygen, whatever the cause, irreversible brain damage occurs within about fifteen minutes.

Why take even a slight chance of this happening to your baby? If you choose a birthing center, please choose one located inside a hospital, next to the labor and delivery department, where – God forbid – if an emergency occurs, precious minutes are not wasted.

Midwives

Midwives can provide an invaluable service to any obstetrical practice. For women desiring a holistic approach to delivery, this is certainly the way to go. In fact, most midwives now practice in hospital settings, utilizing birthing rooms that are designed to make mothers feel at home, but which are only seconds away from help, should an emergency arise.

Virtually all medical equipment and monitors are discreetly hidden in cabinets and closets. Decorative wallpaper covers the once-sterile walls, and designer quilts cover the beds. Sofas and upholstered chairs are there for the comfort of loved ones. Intercoms can be muted, and privacy is absolutely maintained. Unless an emergency arises, hospital staff members stay out of the room.

Marjeta's midwife was trained years ago at a time when midwives sometimes developed a distrust of their obstetrical counterparts. More recent midwifery training programs encourage a more collegiate relationship between the two. These improved relations are important, making midwives more likely to call for consultation earlier in the labor-and-delivery process than in the past.

But despite Marjeta's prolonged rupture of uterine, her midwife did not call for help. Neither her low-grade fever nor her eventual high temperature prompted a call. Incredibly, the midwife did not call for help or even implement electronic fetal heart monitoring when Jana's increased heart rate failed to abate. These were all tremendous risks and warnings that Jana and Marjeta were suffering from some sort of infection, which is always a high-risk situation.

Further, the fact that Marjeta had undergone a C-section with her first birth should have mandated labor and delivery in a hospital setting. Although small (five to seven per 1,000 deliveries), the risk of uterine rupture is very real. Such a rupture can be life-threatening to both mom and baby within minutes. Midwives trained today would not risk allowing a woman with a previous C-section to labor outside a hospital setting.

Women who are considering using a midwife for labor and delivery must have a thorough understanding of their support and backup systems. As mentioned, all midwives must have obstetrical support. Expectant mothers need to know exactly what this entails.

Marjeta's midwife had available obstetrical support, but her philosophy was to access this help only in case of an emergency. The problem was, she did not recognize the emergency as it unfolded, had unfounded confidence in her ability to handle it alone, or chose not to call her obstetrician for some other reason.

If you are planning to use a midwife, you must interview not only her, but also her supporting obstetrician. In such cases, you must use your best judgment and your intuition. What is the nature of the midwife's and obstetrician's comments about each other? Do their attitudes toward each other seem to be mutually admirable or strained?

You should ask your midwife what situations would prompt her to call for a consult. Is she conservative, tending to opt for early consultation? Besides her obstetrical backup, what other support exists in the hospital? Does the facility have in-house physicians at all times, in case the obstetrical backup is unavailable in the event of an emergency?

We support your choice to use a midwife in the case of a normal, healthy pregnancy. But just as we recommend every mother-to-be should thoroughly research her obstetrician, the same applies to her midwife. You should only consider using a midwife who delivers in a hospital setting. When it comes to your well-being and that of your unborn child, we are unabashedly conservative. Some women and some health care providers may be upset by our recommendations. We make no apologies.

Although the vast majority of deliveries are successful, a bad obstetrical outcome can have far-reaching consequences. Besides the obvious maternal or fetal harm, the subsequent stress and guilt can affect family members and all those who interact with the mother. Other children suffer because of the time commitment involved in caring for a disabled child. Marriages and relationships suffer if finger-pointing takes place. What should have been a joyful experience can revert to confusion, pain and sorrow for years to come.

We admonish you to put your baby's safety above all else. That's what you will do once the baby arrives, so why behave any differently while the baby is still in the womb?

CHAPTER 19

What Every Expectant Mother Should Know

Introduction

Babies live and grow inside a fluid-filled sac called the *amniotic cavity*. It gets its name from the membrane in direct contact with the fluid – the amnion.

This membrane is comprised of just a single layer of cells. It has many important functions, not the least of which is to protect the baby from infection. The fluid within the sac is a combination of secretions from the amnion and sterile urine from the baby. An important characteristic of the fluid from the amnion, especially later in pregnancy, is that it has a bacteria-static function. That is, it helps fight any bacteria that may find their way into the amniotic cavity.

The chorion, a thicker membrane that faces the uterine lining, further supports the amnion. Between these two layers is connective tissue that is important in nurturing the membrane.

The exact cause of membrane rupture is not fully understood. Certainly, the area over the cervix is at greatest risk because it is the most poorly supported part of the fluid-filled sac. It is also the place of least blood supply, so the membranes don't receive as much nutrition and become weakened. This part of the membrane is also in closest proximity to the vagina, which is a tremendous source of potential infection.

Normally, the cervix is closed and filled with thick mucus, which prevents vaginal bacteria from ascending to the membranes. However, there are times when the bacteria do reach the membranes and cause localized inflammation, weakening the membranes and leading to eventual rupture.

Premature rupture of membranes (PROM) is defined as rupture that is not followed by the onset of contractions within one hour. When this occurs prior to thirty-seven weeks of gestation (considered term), this condition is called *preterm premature rupture of* membranes (PPROM). Most women at or near term will start labor spontaneously within twenty-four hours.

Diagnosis

Marjeta was awakened by a warm, damp feeling in her vaginal area. This is the classic symptom women feel with membrane rupture. It can range from fluid literally gushing from the vagina to merely a sensation of unusual dampness. The symptoms vary, in part, depending on the size and location of the rupture. A small rupture not located over the cervix can leak only small amounts of fluid intermittently and can be difficult to diagnose. Fortunately, membrane rupture is usually obvious.

Other things may cause vaginal moistness, as well. It's not uncommon for a woman to think membrane rupture has occurred, only to be disproven when tested. Certain vaginal infections can cause an abnormal moist sensation; most are benign and safely treated. An unrealized loss of urine may be the most common cause, especially later in pregnancy. This can occur when lifting, coughing, sneezing, or even just getting up from a chair. Each of these activities increases the pressure on the abdomen and bladder, which in turn can cause a little urine loss. Because the bladder lies at the lower part of the uterus, the baby's kicking or punching in this area is another known cause of urine loss.

If you suspect something is not right, it is best to see your doctor right away. You should never feel foolish asking to be checked for membrane rupture, even if you have done so several times and been found negative. This is especially true if the person performing testing is unfamiliar to you, such as a health care provider at the hospital late at night.

The majority of the time, rupture is obvious, simply by the observation of amniotic fluid coming out through the vagina. Testing can be performed when symptoms are less obvious.

The most common diagnostic tool used is the Nitrazine test. The pH of the vagina is slightly acidic, and that of amniotic fluid is alkaline (basic). Those of you who remember your high school chemistry probably recall performing tests using litmus paper to see whether something had an acidic or basic character. If the paper was red, that meant it was acidic; if it was blue, that meant it had a basic character. The Nitrazine test simply uses a yellow piece of litmus paper to test your vaginal secretions. A paper that turns blue indicates membrane rupture.

This test is about 98 percent effective in detecting ruptured membranes. Probably the most common reason for failure is the failure of the person testing to obtain an adequate sampling from the vagina. Most health care providers test by placing the paper at or just inside the opening of the vagina. This is perfectly adequate as an initial screen; however, it is not adequate if the leak is small, as the amniotic fluid tends to pool in the posterior portion of the vagina.

If the initial Nitrazine test is negative, the provider should next perform a sterile speculum exam. This allows direct observation of the cervix for signs of fluid leakage, as well as a sampling from the posterior part of the vagina, usually obtained with a sterile cotton swab.

If rupture is not visibly obvious, the examiner should wipe the swab on a new piece of Nitrazine and on a glass slide. Whether the Nitrazine is positive or negative, the examiner should wait for the slide to dry and then look at it under a microscope. Because of the salt content in amniotic fluid, when it dries and is examined microscopically, a fern-like pattern is observed. Absence of this pattern is virtually always associated with intact membranes.

Very rarely, the Nitrazine test may be negative, but the signs and symptoms so convincing that the obstetrical provider may want to perform further testing. This is especially true if the mother is at less than thirty-six weeks of gestation. Performing an ultrasound is the simplest method to determine the amount of fluid in the amniotic sac. A normal amount is reassuring that rupture has not occurred, while a decreased amount is more concerning.

If there still remains a question, the provider may resort to doing an amniocentesis (placing a needle through the abdomen into the amniotic cavity) and injecting blue dye into the fluid. A tampon is then inserted into the vagina and left there for eight to twelve hours to see if it stains blue. If not, the membranes are intact.

Management

No matter what the cause, once the amniotic membranes rupture, the risk of infection increases significantly. How far along you are in your pregnancy determines the appropriate management. If you experience PPROM and are at less than thirty-two to thirty-four weeks of gestation, watchful waiting is appropriate because the risk of harm to the baby from prematurity outweighs the risk of infection. This is only true as long as the baby does not become infected and septic.

You will be closely monitored in the hospital for warning signs of early infection. Unfortunately, these signs are non-specific and not always present. Remember, Marjeta felt some mild tenderness in her abdomen and had a low-grade fever. These are both signs of infection, as is an increased heart rate in mom or baby. They mandate an immediate, detailed evaluation, many times leading to antibiotic coverage and delivery of the baby. Although prematurity is a risk in and of itself, when you add sepsis into the picture, it is virtually always a formula for injury to the baby.

Besides temperature and tenderness (deriving from the uterus, felt through the abdomen), the provider will also monitor blood tests closely. Your white blood cell count and a substance called *C-reactive protein* (CRP) are both known markers for infection. A rise in either is an indicator of impending infection. Along with findings of a physical exam, these tests help an obstetrician decide the best course for you and your baby.

Final determinants in case management involve testing the baby. This is done by ultrasound, fetal heart monitoring, and obtaining a sample of the amniotic fluid. A test called a *biophysical profile* measures the amniotic fluid volume, as well as the baby's breathing, movement, and tone. Each category is assigned a score of two, if present, or zero, if absent. Obviously, with ruptured membranes, it is not uncommon to receive a zero for fluid volume, but if the baby is doing well, each of the remaining three categories should be assigned a two.

Of the three remaining categories, fetal breathing is the most important, especially after thirty-two weeks gestation. There is a definite association between absence of fetal breathing and neonatal infection.

The final part of the biophysical profile concerns how the baby's fetal heart rate appears on the EFM tracing. This measure is also assigned a score of zero or two. If the tracing is reactive (two heart rate accelerations of fifteen beats above baseline, each lasting fifteen seconds, within a twenty-minute period), a score of two is assigned. If not, the assessment is zero.

The total score available is ten. If the score is four or less, immediate delivery is almost always indicated. A six means testing should be repeated within twenty-four hours, but even in this case, we recommend you be moved to a labor-and-delivery suite, where fetal monitoring can be conducted continuously and vital signs taken much more frequently, as well as evaluation for tenderness.

Usually, a sample of amniotic fluid can be obtained from the posterior area of your vagina and sent to the lab for testing for phosphatidylglycerol (PG) and the lecithin-sphingomyelin ratio (L/S). These are substances your baby's lungs secrete into the amniotic fluid, but only once the lungs are mature. If testing reveals they are present in significant amounts, delivery should take place soon afterward.

If maternal and fetal testing results are within normal limits, but your baby's lungs are still immature, continued testing should be conducted during the balance of the pregnancy. An ultrasound should be performed twice weekly, and the fetal heart monitoring should be carried out daily. Fetal tachycardia (heart rate above 160) is also a sign of possible infection in your baby. In addition, fluids for testing your baby's lung maturity should be obtained and tested weekly. Furthermore, your temperature should be taken at least three to four times daily, and your blood should be checked daily for signs of infection.

The period between thirty-three and thirty-five weeks of gestation is a gray area for management. At some point during this time, the risk of infection outweighs the risk of prematurity, and delivery is indicated. The closer you get to thirty-five weeks, the lower the threshold for delivery. Very early or unclear signs of infection that may have justified a wait-and-see course at twenty-eight weeks should now mandate a more aggressive delivery plan.

After thirty-five weeks, there is nothing to be gained by waiting. The risk of infection clearly outweighs any concerns about prematurity. The longer you remain undelivered, the greater chance your baby has of becoming infected.

Waiting more than forty-eight hours, as Marjeta's midwife did, is absolutely unacceptable. The risk of infection is less than 10 percent when delivery is accomplished within twenty-four hours of premature rupture of membranes and increases to 40 percent after this time. Although most women go into labor within twenty-four hours of PROM, at this gestational age, waiting any longer than six hours unnecessarily puts your baby at risk. If you haven't started labor by then, medication such as Pitocin should be given to initiate the labor process. (Ideally, labor should be induced as soon as PROM is diagnosed.)

Infection

Introduction

Chorioamnionitis is the medical term used to describe a variety of symptoms found in the presence of infection. Strictly speaking, it means inflammation of the fetal membranes (the chorion and, occasionally, the amnion) and amniotic fluid. It can have severe consequences for both you and your baby.

Although serious long-term complications from chorioamnionitis are rare in the mother, it can lead to endometritis (infection in the uterus), sepsis (infection in the mother's blood) and, very occasionally, death. A combination of antibiotics and delivery (which removes the source of infection) virtually always assures maternal well-being. In the rare event of the mother's death, there are almost always extenuating circumstances, such as treatment having been delayed for an extended time or the presence of conditions causing an abnormally decreased immune response (such as HIV).

Fortunately, chorioamnionitis usually does not cause early-onset neonatal infection (EONI), defined as infection within seventy-two hours of birth. But when present, EONI can have devastating consequences for your baby, especially if treatment is delayed. Therefore, accurately diagnosing and treating chorioamnionitis is paramount for the well-being of both mother and child.

Signs and Symptoms

Risk factors associated with chorioamnionitis include premature labor, PROM, PPROM, rupture of membranes longer than twenty-four hours, a prior history of a preterm birth, and poor maternal nutrition and health. African-American women have been shown to be at greater risk for chorioamnionitis than women of other races. Other associated risks include frequent pelvic exams (especially after ruptured membranes), amniocentesis, meconium, and internal fetal monitoring.

Clinical findings associated with chorioamnionitis include increased maternal temperature, maternal and/or fetal tachycardia, increased white blood cell count and/or C-reactive protein, and uterine tenderness. The presence of two or more of these symptoms is associated with an increased risk of neonatal infection. Remember, Marjeta had both a tender uterus and a fever.

Of all the tests for chorioamnionitis, CRP may be the one performed least often, especially when immediate induction of labor is planned. However, if membrane rupture occurs and immediate delivery is not scheduled, this test should be performed with your routine labs. Like any test results, CRP should not be looked at in isolation; however, it is a very important factor in determining whether chorioamnionitis is present. Levels greater than thirty milligrams per liter indicate the presence of infection.

Causes

Certain aspects of pregnancy protect against infection, but others make you more vulnerable to infection.

Typically, your immune system defends against anything it perceives as foreign. For example, the characteristics of different blood types are expressed as antigens. If your body senses an antigen different from yours, the immune system attempts to destroy the unfamiliar antigens and their source. That is why blood is tested before a transfusion is given; it is important to ensure the antigens match.

Half of your baby's genes come from your partner, so it makes sense that some unfamiliar antigens will be present. Yet, your body doesn't attack your baby. Many factors play into this, one of which is a decrease in your immune response caused by pregnancy. This decrease makes you more susceptible to infection.

As mentioned earlier, your amniotic fluid has bacteria-static capabilities, mainly regulated by a zinc-based compound. As pregnancy progresses, the density and the protection afforded by this compound increases. Obviously, once your membranes rupture, this protection starts to wane. A diet deficient in zinc also decreases the amount of this substance present.

Chorioamnionitis is virtually always caused by bacteria ascending from your vagina into the uterus. The two most common types are E. coli and group B streptococcus. The infection may be mild (involving only the outer chorionic membrane) to severe (possibly even crossing both membranes and entering the umbilical cord and your baby's blood stream). Fortunately, this latter extreme is uncommon.

Prevention and Treatment
Group B strep can be found in more than 40 percent of recto-vaginal cultures at one time or another. It is a known pathogen in newborns; when not treated in a timely manner, it can cause the baby to suffer sepsis, meningitis, and even brain injury or death. As little as a four- to six-hour delay in antibiotic treatment can mean the difference between no permanent injury and serious consequences for the baby, including brain injury and death.

That is why all pregnant women are tested between thirty-five and thirty-seven weeks of gestation. This is done by swabbing the rectum and the front one-third of the vagina. These swabs are then sent for culturing. If you test is positive, you will receive antibiotics during labor to protect both you and your baby. Be aware it takes four hours to get adequate antibiotic levels to your baby, so delivery before this time requires a heightened sensitivity to signs of fetal infection.

You should also be aware that even a negative test does not guarantee the absence of bacteria. The test is only felt to be a reliable indicator for a three- to five-week period because the vagina can become colonized by group B strep bacteria at any time. Another important factor affecting reliability is sampling error. It is extremely important that the culture be taken from the proper locations of your vagina and your rectum. Failure to do so can easily lead to a false-negative result.

Infection of the baby can occur either early, within seventy-two hours of birth, or later, at ten to fourteen days of life. You must be extremely alert to early signs of infection during this time period. Remember, only a few hours' delay in treatment can make all the difference. Lethargy and poor feeding are the two most reliable signs of early infection in your baby. These may be accompanied by either an increased or decreased temperature. Any of these signs require immediate examination. If you did test positive for group B strep, tell the doctor examining your baby without delay.

E. coli is the other common bacteria responsible for EONI. This is a normal bacteria found in the colon and is not cultured for prior to delivery. Proper anogenital hygiene is the best prevention method, but although helpful, it certainly doesn't guarantee your baby won't be exposed during delivery.

Other Infections

Herpes II, which occurs in the genital area, is an extremely common adult infection. Transmission to your baby is never good. It can express itself as disease located only on your baby's skin, eyes and mouth, or it can manifest far more seriously, as meningitis (inflammation of the membranes surrounding the brain). While the former conditions have no long-term serious effects, the latter almost always results in permanent brain injury and/or death.

All herpes viruses live in the nerve ganglions (roots), usually in a dormant state. When they become active, they travel down the nerve, and usually express themselves as visible lesions on the skin, in the area where the virus first gained entry at the time of initial infection. However, the virus can also be shed asymptomatically from your cervix, with or without a lesion on the cervix.

A large percentage of neonatal herpes infections occur in newborns whose mothers have never had a sign or symptom of the disease. This is a disconcerting statistic – one we feel has not been appropriately addressed by the American College of Obstetricians and Gynecologists. Furthermore, women known to have herpes, but with no active lesions, will all test positive by cervical culture at some point during every 100-day period. Although this may not sound significant, it means asymptomatic shedding of the virus occurs on at least three days during the pregnancy of an asymptomatic woman known to have herpes.

A primary infection around the time of delivery is much more dangerous than a recurrent infection. The good news is that intact membranes will almost always protect your baby from infection. The antiviral drugs acyclovir and famciclovir can also virtually eliminate risk to your baby.

Because of the disastrous effects of herpes in the newborn infant, we recommend the following:

- Get your blood tested for herpes early in pregnancy.

- If you test positive or have a known history of herpes, start prophylactic acyclovir or famcyclovir at thirty-six weeks of gestation.

- At the first sign of ruptured membranes, see your doctor immediately to be checked for the presence of lesions. This includes a speculum exam of your cervix.

- If a lesion is present or you have symptoms of an impending infection, delivery should be accomplished by C-section. In the presence of ruptured membranes and/or labor, delivery should be expedited.

- In the absence of a lesion or symptoms, vaginal delivery is safe.

If your baby is exposed to herpes, infection can take as long as two to three weeks to declare itself. Follow the same instructions and diligence outlined for late-onset group B strep, including report-ing your history of herpes to your pediatrician. During the first few months of your child's life, any such history should also be reported to others who have occasion to provide health care to your child, such as an emergency room physician.

Chicken pox and herpes zoster also stem from the herpes family. This class of viruses is called *varicella-zoster virus* (VZV).

Herpes zoster (shingles) is a late complication of chickenpox. It is characterized by very painful lesions appearing along different areas on the skin, called *dermatomes*, supplied by the nerves in which the virus lives. Maternal outbreaks of shingles are not known to cause malformations to the fetus.

On the other hand, a maternal outbreak of chicken pox can have serious effects on you and your baby. If you are considering pregnancy and don't know whether you have had chicken pox or the vaccine for chicken pox, you should be tested prior to trying to conceive. If you are not immune to the virus (never had the disease or the vaccine), then you should be vaccinated at least four weeks prior to trying to get pregnant.

If you are already pregnant and are unsure of your immune status with regard to chicken pox, you should be tested with your first set of labs. Be sure to tell your provider you are unsure of your status and request this testing, as it is not routinely done. If you are found to be susceptible, you absolutely must avoid any possible exposure to a person suspected of having chicken pox – typically, a child. The virus tends to be prevalent in the late winter and early spring, so be particu-larly careful during those times.

A person infected with chicken pox sheds the virus for up to three weeks. A susceptible person exposed to the virus in a household has more than a 90 percent chance of catching the disease. If you are exposed at work, this rate drops to approximately 10 to 20 percent.

It is also extremely important to be tested when you have chicken pox during pregnancy. If you have the disease during weeks eight to twenty of your pregnancy, your baby has more than a 10 percent chance of also being infected. Although the risk of your baby becoming infected during this time is small, if infected, the baby's risks are potentially serious, including scars, limb problems, eye problems, poor growth (intrauterine growth restriction, or IUGR), an abnormally small head size (microcephaly), delayed development, and/or cognitive impairment.

Fortunately, tests are available to help determine whether your baby is affected. Frequent ultrasounds should be performed to ensure your baby is growing properly, and your baby's extremities should be checked to ensure they are not affected. You should also see a high-risk obstetrician to discuss cordocentesis, a test in which a needle is passed through your abdomen and uterus into the umbilical cord to sample your baby's blood. The blood is then tested to discern whether an intrauterine infection has occurred.

If you have chickenpox around the time of delivery, your baby has more than a 40 percent chance of becoming infected. This is very important, as a newborn infant is not able to fight the infection well, and the mortality (death) rate for infected babies exceeds 30 percent. If there is any chance of infection, both you and your baby should receive varicella-zoster immune globulin (VZIG). Although VZIG does not decrease the chance of your baby becoming infected, it has been shown to decrease the severity of the infection. You should receive the injection because pregnancy and adulthood both increase the risk of the severity of the infection, which can be life-threatening.

Cytomegalovirus (CMV) is another member of the herpes virus group. Most women are immune to it, but a significant percentage of women are not, especially Caucasians. Fortunately, even if you are not immune, exposure during pregnancy causes maternal infection less than 4 percent of the time.

Unfortunately, you may have absolutely no symptoms of a CMV infection. If you do, they typically last from three to twelve weeks and include low-grade fever, malaise, swollen glands, muscle aches, and sore throat. The CMV virus is passed through the saliva, urine, semen, and cervical mucous of infected persons. Children, especially those in day care, most commonly host and transmit the virus.

In women who become infected with CMV for the first time during pregnancy, transmission of the infection to their babies occurs in 25 to 75 of cases. Fortunately, babies experience severe complications only ten to 15 percent of the time. However, when they do occur, the devastating effects can include hearing loss, blindness, microcephaly, and profound mental retardation.

Should you be diagnosed with a primary infection, testing of the amniotic fluid and blood through the umbilical cord can help determine the risk of infection to your baby. Serial ultrasound exams should also be performed to further delineate early problems. Even if you are immune (previously exposed and infected with CMV), there is a small risk the virus could become reactivated during pregnancy. Fortunately, the effects on your baby are rarely serious, with less than 1 percent developing mental retardation.

Toxoplasmosis is a protozoan that is found in mammals. It is rare, affecting less than 1 percent of all babies born. However, it can have serious effects on your baby at any time during pregnancy. Many women are immune to this disease. Unfortunately, if you do acquire it during pregnancy, you may have no symptoms. When symptoms are present, they commonly include swollen lymph nodes in the neck and a general feeling of tiredness and malaise. Should you have either of these symptoms, get tested right away, as medications are available to help protect your baby.

Preventing infection is the best approach and is relatively easy. The two most common modes of infection are eating undercooked meat and exposure to cat feces.

If you eat meat during your pregnancy, it should be cooked to well-done – to a temperature of 65 degrees Celcius/149 degrees Fahrenheit – to eliminate any risk of infection. The toxoplasmosis organisms can also be destroyed by freezing, but your freezer at home likely doesn't achieve low enough temperatures to accomplish this. Because industrial freezers do, meat that has been frozen by the supplier is safest.

Finally, if you handle raw meat, be sure to wash your hands and all utensils thoroughly after doing so.

If you own a cat, you should never change the litter box; someone else in the household must assume that responsibility. The box must be located in an isolated area, and you must avoid going near it. The cysts that carry this infection are very stable to temperature, and only those over 60 degrees Celcius/140 degrees Fahrenheit will destroy them. Someone besides you should disinfect the litter box regularly by boiling it in water for about five minutes.

The last disease we will talk about, fifth disease, is caused by the parvovirus B-19. It gets its name from being the fifth disease in children that causes a red rash. Typically, the rash appears on the face – bright red, almost as if the child was recently slapped – and spreads to the arms and chest, sparing the palms of the hands.

As with other diseases we've discussed, more than 60 percent of you have been exposed to this disease prior to your pregnancy and are immune to it. It is transmitted through saliva and mucous, and is most frequently acquired from close proximity to infected pre-school and elementary-age children.

This virus almost always causes symptoms, including rash, fever, swollen glands and lymph nodes, and mild arthritic symptoms in the hands, wrists, and knees.

Exposure after twenty-one to twenty-four weeks of gestation rarely poses a risk to your baby. Prior to this stage, it may cause problems such as low blood count (anemia), damage to your baby's heart, or miscarriage. The risk is greatest (about 20 percent) during the first trimester, decreasing to about 6 percent by twenty weeks.

Certain blood tests can confirm or eliminate suspicion of infection in the mother. If the infection is confirmed, serial ultrasound exams will reveal whether your baby has contracted and suffered any consequences of the disease.

CHAPTER 20

Questions to Ask Your Midwife

- Do you deliver in a hospital? If the answer is *no*, we recommend finding one who does.

- What arrangements have you made for physician backup in the event it becomes necessary? (Insist on meeting with the physician, and make sure your prenatal records are provided to them throughout your pregnancy.)

- How long does it take your backup physician to get to the hospital when called?

- Does the hospital have in-house obstetricians twenty-four hours a day, seven days a week, in the case of an emergency?

- Will you use a fetal monitor while I am in labor?

Topics to Discuss Regarding Infections

(For Your Midwife and Obstetrician)

- If you are unaware of any exposure to herpes II, ask to be tested with your first set of prenatal labs.

- If you test positive for herpes II, ask to receive the prophylactic acyclovir or famcyclovir, starting at thirty-six weeks.

- During labor, ask to be informed immediately if any sign of infection is present in either you or your baby.

- If you suspect your membranes have ruptured, ask for both the Nitrazine test and the fern test to confirm or dispel doubt.

- If you have any signs of a viral illness during pregnancy, especially in the first trimester, ask to receive a TORCH panel, which tests for toxoplasmosis; rubella, which is always tested for in the beginning of pregnancy; CMV; and herpes.

PART VII

Your Baby Should Not Have To Shoulder The Problems of Shoulder Dystocia

CHAPTER 21

Brandi's Story

It is late in the afternoon on a Thursday. Thoroughly fed up and exhausted, Brandi drives to her obstetrician's office for a scheduled appointment. Almost thirty-nine weeks pregnant, her prenatal course has been unremarkable from a medical perspective, but the last couple of weeks have drained her. She has added an excessive amount of weight to her already-stocky frame; at five feet, four inches tall, she has ballooned to 227 pounds. Brandi wants her baby delivered now. She feels she simply cannot take this pregnancy any longer.

As she pulls into the parking lot, Brandi's mind drifts back to the day she learned she was pregnant. She was so utterly filled with joy. Brandi remembers how elated her husband, Anthony, was when she told him, and how ecstatic and supportive their parents were at the news. As she recalls those wonderful experiences, a smile spreads across her face – regardless of how miserable she feels now.

Brandi continues to smile as she relives special moments in her pregnancy – the positive news that came with each of her lab tests and ultrasounds, her joy at hearing her baby's heartbeat for the first time, at learning her baby was perfectly formed, and hearing she was having a baby girl. *A daughter,* she had thought at the time. *Just what I hoped for.*

Brandi thinks back happily on the long, lively debates she and Anthony had about what to name their little girl before finally settling on *Kara*.

But as she turns off the engine and struggles to wriggle out from behind the steering wheel, Brandi's smile disappears. Just this small effort saps her remaining energy, and snaps her back to her current reality – she is excessively overweight, bloated, beyond uncomfortable, and exhausted by even the easiest tasks. *And it's time for another pelvic exam. Great.*

She knows the exams are necessary, especially during the last few weeks of pregnancy, but she can't help but wonder: *Why do they have to be so uncomfortable?*

As she has done so many times before, Brandi disrobes, slips into a gown, and climbs onto the examining table with the help of a nurse, who guides her feet into stirrups. Her doctor begins the exam. This time is no different: Brandi's vagina feels extremely tight, and the exam is almost painful. She can't help but wonder: *When the time comes for delivery, will my baby be able to squeeze through?*

"Why are these exams so uncomfortable?" she asks. "Why do I feel so tight?" Brandi's obstetrician reassures her that what she's experiencing is common during first pregnancies, explaining that nervousness and being unable to relax during the exams are to blame. Naturally, Brandi assumes her doctor is correct. *He knows best,* she thinks. *After all, he's a doctor with years and years of experience.*

Brandi's doctor tells her she is dilated to three centimeters, and he will induce labor tomorrow. She is so excited and relieved that she has trouble focusing as her doctor explains the induction process.

As she heads for her car a short while later, she is no longer thinking about being exhausted. Soon, she is home and sharing the good news with her husband and family.

The sun rises on a new day, and a big one it will be. Brandi's bags are packed, and soon she's on her way to the hospital. She arrives at 6:00 a.m., as instructed. Like all first-time mothers, she is nervous as she walks through the hospital doors. But those jitters disappear as she settles into the birthing room and meets her nurse, who is pleasant and reassuring. An IV is started, and she is connected to an electronic fetal monitor, and instantly sees Kara's heartbeat appear on a monitor.

Soon, Brandi's doctor arrives to perform another pelvic exam; however, this one will be a bit different. The OB reminds Brandi he is about to use the instrument in his hand to rupture her bag of water to speed up the delivery process. The exam proceeds without problem, other than being even more uncomfortable than usual.

Next, the doctor administers the labor-inducing drug, Pitocin, which starts Brandi's contractions. As they intensify, she is given pain medication that relaxes her and even allows her to doze off for a few hours. But when the pain medication wears off, she is awakened by almost unbearably painful contractions.

The doctor comes in to see Brandi without delay. He examines her, finding her cervix has dilated to five centimeters. She must reach ten centimeters before she is fully dilated and can begin pushing. The doctor orders an epidural, and, once dosed, Brandi experiences almost instant pain relief. She nods off again.

Several more hours pass before Brandi's obstetrician re-examines her. For the first time, he seems a bit concerned. She has not progressed toward delivery as quickly as he would have liked and expected. The external monitor currently recording Brandi's contractions measures their frequency and duration, but not their strength. The OB tells her he is going to use an intra-uterine pressure catheter (IUPC) to measure the strength of her contractions. He inserts a thin, soft tube filled with water into her uterus and connects it to a monitor. Measurement of contraction strength is now possible.

The measurement shows the contractions are not as strong as they should be, and Brandi's doctor orders the Pitocin to be increased.

Later in the afternoon, Brandi's OB performs another pelvic exam, which showed her dilated to nine centimeters. The nurse informs Brandi she is now at nine centimeters. However, Brandi's relief is cut short when the nurse adds, "There is a 'but.' Your baby has not descended very far down the birth canal. There is no reason to be concerned, as this often happens, especially with a first pregnancy." Reassured, Brandi relaxes once again.

Another two hours pass. Brandi's cervix is finally ten centimeters dilated, and it's time to start pushing. The obstetrical nurse emphasizes she must give it all she's got, explaining the baby has only moved slightly farther down the pelvis since the last exam. In terms of her position in the birth canal, there is still a long way to travel.

Thanks to the epidural, Brandi is well-rested and feels up to the task. She is energized and excited about the prospect of soon meeting little Kara. With Anthony by her side, helping with her breathing, she bears down.

After about an hour and a half of pushing, Brandi's doctor does another pelvic exam. Despite the increased Pitocin and Brandi's strong pushing, Kara has barely budged.

It is approximately 7:30 on a Friday night.

The OB offers a solution to speed delivery along. "To facilitate delivery, I could use a vacuum device, which has a suction cup that would be placed on Kara's head. Your daughter should be in your arms within a few minutes from the time I apply it," her doctor says.

Just yesterday, Brandi wanted to give birth as soon as possible, but she now prefers to finish the process without the use of a vacuum extractor. After all, her nurse told her it can take up to three hours for a first-time mother to deliver once pushing begins. Only half that time has elapsed.

When she expresses her preference, her doctor seems displeased and leaves the room abruptly. She wonders whether his reaction is influenced by the fact that it is a Friday night, but she says nothing, giving him the benefit of the doubt.

Brandi struggles through another half-hour of pushing, and her doctor returns for yet another pelvic exam. When it reveals baby Kara has barely moved, he says it is time to move on to the vacuum. He presents it not as an option, but as the only course of action available. Following a brief discussion, Brandi agrees. Once again, she accepts that her doctor knows best.

Very quickly, Brandi is placed in stirrups for delivery. Her nurse is at one side and her husband at the other.

A suction cup is inserted into the birth canal and placed on baby Kara's head. Suction is applied, and one pull with the vacuum is attempted. The baby doesn't budge. Suction is applied a second time, and another pull is attempted. Still no movement. After a third try fails, at the doctor's direction, the nurse applies pressure high on Brandi's belly, and Brandi exerts all the pushing force she can muster.

Calmly, the doctor announces, "The baby's head is out." But scarcely a moment later, the OB's bearing and tone change dramatically. "The baby is stuck!" he shouts. His sense of pride and accomplishment is rapidly replaced by panic. The nurse also appears to be extremely concerned. Anthony, who began looking a bit pale after the first pull, blanches with fear.

The nurse yells orders to Brandi's husband. "Grab your wife's leg and pull it all the way back on her abdomen!" He gathers himself and does as told. The nurse maneuvers Brandi's other leg in the same way. Brandi can feel her doctor reaching deep inside her, trying to get Kara out. He stands in an attempt to get better leverage and exert more pressure. It doesn't work.

Brandi desperately searches her doctor's eyes. They seem to scream uncertainty. In fact, the man she has trusted so completely now seems virtually paralyzed. In the next instant, he is pulling again, this time on Kara's head. Brandi feels she is being dragged off the table. At the top of her lungs, she yells, "Is my baby alright?" There is no immediate answer, but within moments, Kara is delivered.

When Brandi hears her baby girl cry, she is overcome with relief. Finally, the nurse assures her the baby is fine. She takes Kara to the bassinet, cleans and swaddles her, and delivers her into Brandi's

PATIENTS' RIGHTS AND DOCTORS' WRONGS®

waiting arms. Despite the mind-numbing fright, everything seems to have turned out well.

A short time later, the nurse takes Kara to the nursery. About an hour has passed when Brandi's obstetrician meekly pushes open her door and asks if she is awake. "I need to speak with you."

Suddenly, Brandi is wide awake, sensing something is very wrong. Clearly, the doctor is nervous. Before he can say anything, she asks, "Is Kara okay?"

"Not entirely," he replies. "Kara is not moving her left arm or hand. It appears some of the nerves on the left side of her neck were stretched while we were doing everything we could to complete the delivery after she got stuck on the way out. However, the good news is this should only be temporary. Within about six months, all should be fine."

Tragically, that was wishful thinking. Three and a half years, two nerve transplant surgeries, and months of physical therapy later, Kara still doesn't have normal use of her injured arm and hand. She can hardly bend her elbow at all, and when she does, she often cries out in pain. Doctors tell Brandi and Anthony there is not much more they can do.

CHAPTER 22

What Went Wrong and Why

What is Shoulder Dystocia?

Shoulder dystocia occurs when one of the baby's shoulders gets stuck behind the pubic bone during vaginal delivery, or in rare cases, becomes lodged posteriorly in the hollow of the sacrum. Essentially, the head has delivered, but the rest of the body is stuck. If proper maneuvers are performed, the baby will not be harmed.

Brandi's obstetrician committed numerous errors. He failed to perform adequate pelvimetry (evaluation of the size of an expectant mother's bony pelvis) and ignored obvious warning signs (Brandi's height and weight, as well as prolonged labor and failed descent of Kara's head). He failed to anticipate the possibility of shoulder dystocia and have adequate staff in the room. Additionally, the OB used the vacuum inappropriately. (Kara's head had not descended to a safe point, and Brandi's labor had not progressed in a normal fashion.) He applied traction to Kara's head and failed to perform the correct maneuvers designed to complete a safe delivery, once shoulder dystocia was recognized.

Brandi didn't have an understanding of these matters until well after the fact, when it was too late to help her daughter. If her obstetrician had concerns about whether her baby would "fit," he never expressed them. Brandi was raised in a rural area and taught by her parents to trust, respect and not question doctors. She now knows she must take a different approach with her obstetrical care and other health care, as well. She wants others to learn from her experience, so they don't have to learn the hard way, as she did.

Under no circumstances should you allow any member of the obstetrical team to pull on your baby's head. Pulling excessively on your baby's head causes the nerves traveling through your baby's neck (known as the *brachial plexus*) to be needlessly stretched. With too much force, injury occurs. Moreover, pulling is absolutely not necessary to effectuate delivery.

Caught by Surprise

Shoulder dystocia is among the most common delivery complications. Fortunately, it is usually mild and easily remedied without injuring the baby. However, it is an obstetrical emergency, and severe dystocia is one of the most frightening complications an obstetrician faces. That's probably why many injuries occur – the doctor panics and pulls too hard on the baby's head in an effort to expedite delivery.

When shoulder dystocia occurs, the baby must be delivered quickly to avoid suffering brain damage from lack of oxygen. In this context, *quickly* means within four to five minutes of the baby's head being delivered and the shoulder becoming stuck. This amount of leeway is available to safely complete delivery, as long as the baby has not exhibited significant signs of being inadequately oxygenated prior to the delivery of the head.

Sometimes, in emergency situations, health care providers – like all of us – sense they have much less time to act than they actually do, and they panic. Only one minute may have passed, but it can seem like an eternity. That perception can be dangerous.

That's what happened in Brandi's case. Kara was fine before the delivery of her head. Her obstetrician easily had about five minutes to deliver her safely. He also had time to bring in extra help to ensure maneuvers were performed appropriately. But Brandi's doctor and nurse panicked. They didn't get the extra help they needed, and most importantly, they failed to perform the one maneuver that almost certainly would have delivered Kara safely.

If there is any risk of your baby being large in size or large in relation to your pelvic size, it is imperative you discuss with your health care providers what will occur in the event of shoulder dystocia. This discussion should include your doctor, the nurses caring for you, and a family member who will be in the birthing room with you.

Injury can also occur following shoulder dystocia due to a physician's or nurse's lack of knowledge or experience. In the last few years, technologically advanced simulation has become available to allow doctors-in-training to gain experience that mimics real-life shoulder dystocia cases. This simulation permits hands-on training without using first patients as guinea pigs. Health care providers who have used this method have been found to be well-prepared to face a real shoulder dystocia emergency. Prior to development of this technology, health care providers often lacked hands-on experience to deal with the complication because it was a circumstance that occurred only infrequently.

In obstetrics, when discussing the likelihood of a vaginal delivery, we talk about "the three Ps" – power, passage and passenger. The first "P" refers to the strength of your contractions; if there is any question about whether your contractions are strong enough, it can be easily answered by the placement of an intrauterine pressure catheter. The second and third refer to the size of your pelvis and the size of your baby, respectively. Be sure you discuss all three "Ps" with your provider.

Obviously, the power of your contractions won't be known until labor begins, but the second two "Ps" can be addressed early in your pregnancy, as well as shortly before or soon after you go into labor. If you suspect you are at risk for this serious complication, we recommend having a statement placed in your chart similar to the example provided in Chapter Twenty-Four.

CHAPTER 23

What Every Expectant Mother Should Know About Shoulder Dystocia

Understanding the Injury

The brachial plexus is a network of nerves that emanate from the upper part of the spine (C5-8, T1) and travel to the shoulder, through the neck, down the arm, and into the hand. Brachial plexus injuries occur when these nerves are damaged. Symptoms may vary from simple loss of sensation over portions of the arm to complete paralysis of the arm, shoulder and hand. There are four types or degrees of injuries.

The most severe is an avulsion, which occurs when the nerve roots are literally torn from their origin at the spine. The second-most severe is rupture, in which the nerve itself is torn, but its attachment at the spine is preserved. Neuroma is third in terms of severity, with the torn nerve healing improperly and forming scar tissue. The least-severe degree of injury is neuropraxia, in which the nerve is stretched, like taffy or bubble gum, without actually tearing.

The resulting injury (called *Erb's palsy* if the upper nerves are involved or *Klumpke's palsy* if the lower nerves are harmed) varies from temporary loss of use of parts of the child's arm or hand, to mild clumsiness in their grip, to total loss of use of the arm, hand and shoulder. If the injury is mild, it may heal over time, but as the severity of the injury increases, permanent impairment becomes more likely. When permanent use of the injured limb is lost, disfigurement of the limb will occur. Surgery may be necessary, and there is usually much pain associated with the inevitable contractures and muscle-wasting over a lifetime.

If it sounds horrible, it is. Thankfully, only about 10 percent of brachial plexus injuries are permanent. With aggressive physical therapy, most resolve within six to eighteen months.

Risk Factors
Although risk factors are identifiable, except for maternal diabetes and macrosomia (a particularly large baby), the American Congress of Obstetricians and Gynecologists takes the self-serving attitude that their predictive value is not high enough to be used in a clinical setting. Your obstetrician will probably tell you the same story, but don't accept it. There are a number of warning signs, including ones that even ACOG acknowledges exist, and to ignore them makes no sense at all. As the number of the following risk factors increases in your pregnancy, so does the risk of shoulder dystocia and injury to your baby:

- Excessive maternal weight gain of more than forty pounds.

- Maternal weight greater than 200 pounds, especially if you are not very tall. This not only puts your baby at risk for excessive weight gain, but also makes it difficult for your obstetrical care provider to accurately estimate your baby's size. If you are in this category, ultrasound exams must be performed to more accurately document your baby's size.

- Gestational diabetes (the type acquired during pregnancy), especially if is poorly controlled.

- Contracted pelvis. This refers to the bony structure of your pelvis through which your baby must travel. Obviously, the size and shape of the pelvis varies among women. By performing a thorough vaginal exam, your provider should be able to roughly assess not only the size of your pelvis, but also the size baby you should be able to deliver vaginally. As in Brandi's case, shoulder dystocia often occurs because of factors other than a large baby. This is certainly one of them, and should be evaluated and discussed at the time of your first pelvic exam.

- Fundal height (the distance between the top of your pubic bone and the top of your uterus, or womb) measures two or more centimeters greater than your gestational age. For example, if your fundal height is thirty-two centimeters and you are twenty-eight weeks pregnant, you are at increased risk. However, a significant discrepancy between fundal height and gestational age may be attributable to something other than a large baby. A sideways or breech position of your baby in the womb, the presence of an excessive amniotic fluid, or carrying twins might explain the disparity.

- Pregnancy that continues past your due date.

- Abnormalities of the active stage of labor (the period during which dilation from four to ten centimeters occurs). Dilatation should progress at approximately one centimeter per hour. If you fail to progress at this pace, your doctor or midwife and nurse should be wary.

- Prolonged second stage of labor, otherwise known as the pushing stage (more than one hour for a second-time mother and more than two hours for a first-time mother). If you have an epidural, each time period may well be extended by about an hour. In that event, there would be about three hours of pushing in first pregnancies and about two hours in subsequent pregnancies.

- Inadequate descent of your baby's head. During labor, your baby will gradually move through your pelvis until eventual delivery. When your doctor or nurse examines you every few hours, part of that exam involves evaluating the location of your baby's head in relation to bony prominences felt through the vaginal wall. These bony parts are called the *ischial spines*. When the top of your baby's head is at the level of the spines, that is called *zero (0) station*. Progress is measured in centimeters above and below zero station. The three centimeters above zero station are assigned negative or minus values (-1, -2 and -3), indicating the baby is still high in the birth canal. As the baby moves downward, its position changes from -3 to -2 to -1, zero station, and then +1, +2, +3, +4, and +5. When your baby reaches +5 station, delivery is imminent. If your baby stays at the same station for one to two hours, especially during the late active phase and pushing, serious consideration should be given to delivery by C-section.

- The need to use a vacuum or forceps. Never allow either of these to be used unless your baby is at least at +3 station and, preferably, even farther down the birth canal. As your baby passes through the pelvis, its shoulders gradually rotate and compress, which allows passage under the pubic bone. Vacuum and forceps speed up this process, sometimes too fast, so adequate rotation does not occur, and the shoulder becomes entrapped.

- Previous delivery of a large baby (heavier than eight and one-half pounds).

- A history of a prior shoulder dystocia in one of your deliveries.

Prevention

Some of these risk factors are known prior to the time an expectant mother goes into labor. If you have any of them in your pregnancy, you must have an ultrasound performed prior to the onset of labor (preferably, between thirty-seven and thirty-eight weeks) to estimate your baby's weight (estimated fetal weight or EFW).

Late in pregnancy, however, the margin of error for estimating your baby's weight by this method can be as much as a pound and a half. Most EFWs are given in grams. There are 454 grams in one pound. So an EFW of 4,000 grams could mean your baby weighs as little as 3,300 grams (seven and a half pounds) or as much as 4,700 grams (ten and a half pounds).

Over the years, ACOG has systematically increased the fetal weight at which a C-section should be offered. It now stands at 4,500 grams for diabetic mothers and 5,000 grams for non-diabetic mothers. By the way, 5,000 grams is greater than eleven pounds. Mothers are usually not counseled until the baby's weight reaches 5,000 grams, but as we have pointed out, there is a large margin of error. A 4,300-gram EFW could well indicate an eleven-pound baby.

Added to this equation is the fact that, after about thirty-five weeks, babies gain 200 to 300 grams of weight per week. So an estimate of 4,000 grams at thirty-seven weeks indicates the baby will weigh more than 4,600 grams at thirty-nine weeks, or full-term.

Many obstetricians follow ACOG guidelines. Unfortunately, the purpose of those guidelines seems to be more about protecting physicians during litigation than about promoting patient safety. A 1999 study, which many seem to have forgotten, showed a fetal abdominal circumference of greater than thirty-five centimeters (measured during an ultrasound exam) was 93 percent predictive of macrosomia, or an abnormally large baby. A second study demonstrated a difference between abdominal diameter and head diameter of 2.6 centimeters or greater in diabetic mothers was highly sensitive and predictive of shoulder dystocia. The ACOG guidelines mention neither. It is imperative to ask your provider about these measurements when reviewing your ultrasound report.

If macrosomia is suspected, it is absolutely necessary to discuss this with your obstetrician. If the EFW is anywhere near 4,000 grams, be sure to follow these steps:

Talk with your obstetrician before labor begins.

- Discuss the risks and benefits of delivering vaginally as opposed to by C-section, as those risks pertain to your individual case. You may have a sense, based on experience or instinct, as to whether the EFW is on the low or high side, and your doctor will certainly have an opinion.

- Agree that under no circumstances will forceps or vacuum be used; your baby must be delivered naturally or by C-section.

- Agree that a C-section will be performed if your labor deviates from (a) the amount of time expected for you to dilate to ten centimeters (plotted by your doctor as something called the *labor curve*) or (b) the amount of time within which delivery is expected to be completed after you start pushing.

- Discuss the use of Pitocin. While it may be perfectly fine to resort to Pitocin, any significant deviation from the normal labor curve should be a sign to move to a C- section.

- If you are delivering vaginally, be sure the appropriate personnel are in the delivery room. At a minimum, two labor-and-delivery nurses should be present, as well as nursery personnel trained in neonatal resuscitation.

- Most importantly, ensure that if shoulder dystocia occurs, no traction will be applied to your baby's head, except in the rare circumstance it is needed as a life-saving procedure.

Just as there are known prenatal risk factors for shoulder dystocia, others can develop for the first time during labor. There are three stages of labor and delivery:

- The first stage of labor extends from the onset of labor until the time you reach full dilation. This stage is further divided into the *latent* phase and the *active* phase.

  o The latent phase in a first-time mother extends from the onset of labor until four centimeters of dilation. In a repeat mother, the latent phase is deemed to last until the mother reaches five centimeters' dilation. This can take anywhere from a few hours to a couple of days. It has little significance in predicting shoulder dystocia.

  o The active phase of labor begins once the four- or five-centimeter mark is reached. During this stage, you should dilate a minimum of one centimeter per hour (from five or six hours up to as many as ten hours). Occasionally, your contractions may not be strong enough, and Pitocin may be required to help. Even in this situation, any time you fall more than two hours behind schedule, a C-section should be seriously considered.

- The second stage of labor is also known as the *pushing stage*. If it is your first time attempting vaginal delivery without an epidural, delivery should occur within two hours; if you have delivered vaginally before, it should occur within about one hour. If you receive epidural anesthesia, these times are extended to three hours and two hours, respectively. That's because the anesthetic effect of the epidural dulls your sensation, which can make your pushing less effective.

We must stress that the time for delivery during the second stage is somewhat arbitrary and assumes your baby is descending adequately. If this is not occurring on a timely basis, your physician should begin preparations for a possible C-section. You should not allow the time periods given for these important events to pass without your health care team's moving toward a Caesarean delivery.

- The third stage of labor is the period extending from delivery of your baby until delivery of the placenta. Obviously, this stage has no bearing on the topic of shoulder dystocia.

When Shoulder Dystocia Occurs

Three maneuvers, when done correctly, will relieve virtually all shoulder dystocia without injury to your baby. The purpose of the first two is to enlarge the space through which the baby has to pass. An episiotomy enlarges the vaginal opening, and hyper-flexing the legs back onto the abdomen (called *McRobert's procedure*) enlarges the space between the public bone and the sacrum.

The third and most important maneuver, by far, is the application of supra-pubic pressure. This option should be discussed with your obstetrician prior to labor and with the entire delivery team after your labor begins. When supra-pubic pressure is applied correctly, it will release virtually any baby's entrapped shoulder. Here's how it is carried out:

- Your bed should be lowered below the waist level of the person applying the pressure in order to gain leverage and exert the necessary force. Pressure should be applied downward at a forty-five-degree angle to rotate the shoulder and push it below the pubic bone.

- If necessary, the person applying the pressure should use the weight of his or her body to exert enough force to complete the rotation and release.

- Under no circumstances should fundal pressure (pushing on your uterus at a level above your navel) ever be used. This will only worsen the entrapment by pushing your baby's shoulder tighter against your pubic bone.

In the unlikely event these first three methods fail, extraordinary measures may be tried to release your baby's shoulder. They include:

- The *Woods corkscrew* or *Reuben corkscrew*. The doctor places a hand in the vagina against either the anterior or posterior aspect of the baby's shoulder. An attempt is then made to sweep or rotate the baby in a clockwise or counterclockwise fashion to release the shoulder. The name of the procedure depends on the direction the shoulder is rotated.

- The *posterior arm sweep*. When the anterior shoulder is entrapped, an attempt may be made to deliver the posterior arm and shoulder first. If successful, it will then enable the anterior shoulder to drop and be released.

- The *Zavenelli maneuver*. Very rarely, and usually only as a life-saving procedure, the doctor pushes the baby's head back into the vagina and then performs an emergency C-section.

CHAPTER 24

Proposed Letter for Obstetrical Team's Signature

If you suspect your baby is at high risk for shoulder dystocia, we recommend signing a letter similar to the one below and having it placed in your doctor's and hospital chart.

To my attending obstetrician and primary nursing staff:

Re:Shoulder Dystocia

I understand I have certain risk factors that could possibly lead to shoulder dystocia at the time of my delivery. I have discussed this at length with my primary obstetrician. I understand all the potential risks, consequences and options. I have elected a trial of vaginal delivery, with the following stipulations:

1. Forceps and vacuum will not be used. If I am unable to deliver vaginally, a C-section will be performed.

2. Once my cervix becomes five centimeters dilated, if this is my first delivery and I have not reached full dilation (ten centimeters) within five to seven hours, a C-section will be

performed. If this is not my first vaginal delivery, a C-section will be performed if I am not fully dilated within four to six hours.

3. During my pushing stage, I will be kept current as to the progress in the descent of my baby's head. After one hour, my attending physician will examine me, and we will discuss my progress and the safest course of action. This will occur again thirty minutes later, if I have not delivered. If I still have not given birth two hours after the onset of the pushing phase of labor, I wish to proceed to C-section. However, if I have been receiving epidural pain relief, these periods maybe extended by one hour, following a discussion with me and obtaining my agreement at that time.

4. When it is time for me to deliver vaginally, in addition to my doctor, at least two labor-and-delivery nurses and a nursery team will be present in the room.

5. If shoulder dystocia is encountered, no traction will be applied to my baby's head. Trained nurses should be holding and managing my legs at this point. My bed should be lowered below the waist level of the shortest nurse. At this point, my legs should be flexed well back on my abdomen, and pressure should be applied just above my pubic bone and to my baby's shoulder so as to first rotate my baby's shoulder to the left or right, and then downwards to allow it to pass under the pubic bone. This should be done in a slow, deliberate manner, using my health care provider's body weight, if necessary.

6. I am not opposed to an episiotomy, should it be deemed necessary to safely deliver my baby.

_____

Signature and Date

I have read and agree to the above plan of care:

_____

Health Care Provider

_____

Health Care Provider

NOTE: All maneuvers covered above have not been included in this letter because, when performed properly, the maneuvers described in this sample letter virtually always work. Furthermore, if this plan is followed without successfully bringing about delivery, you would then be dealing with an emergency that requires immediate action by your obstetrician.

Hopefully, you never have to face this situation, but if this complication develops, making your desires known to your care providers and making sure they are prepared to honor them can be invaluable.

PART VIII

Surgical Emergencies During Pregnancy

CHAPTER 25

Beth's Story

(As Told from the Perspective of Dr. Giles H. Manley)
Early Friday morning, Beth awakes to a wave of nausea. She is twenty weeks pregnant with her second child. Although she experienced some morning sickness during her first trimester, this seems different somehow. But Beth is a mother and a schoolteacher, and a lot of people are counting on her. She resolves to push past the sick feeling and get on with her day. *Once I get up and start moving around, I'll be fine,* she thinks.

But as she rolls out of bed, she is hit by a sudden, sharp pain that almost takes her to the floor. After a few seconds, slowly, gingerly, she manages to straighten up. The pain slowly eases as she catches her breath. Her brow damp with perspiration, Beth steps into the shower. As the warm water washes over her body, she begins to feel better.

Still, Beth is concerned. She has had one child, and she has read all the literature about pregnancy. This just doesn't seem normal. She considers calling her obstetrician, but it is still very early, and she is feeling a little better. She consoles herself with the fact that she has his cell phone number. If she starts feeling worse, she can call him right away.

Beth has a big day ahead. It's the last day of school before summer break. Her fifth-grade class gets out at noon, and she has heard through the grapevine they will be throwing her a surprise baby shower. *It's so sweet of them to do that. I just can't disappoint them.*

But the last hour of the morning is tough. Beth's nausea is intensifying, and the pain in her lower abdomen is worsening. She wipes her forehead, as she again begins to perspire. The instant her class is over, she calls her obstetrician – who happens to be me. I tell her to come to the office immediately.

Beth has been my patient for five years, and I know her very well. I saw her through the birth of her first child and also through a prior surgery. She is not a complainer, and the uneasiness in her voice concerns me.

My concern deepens when she arrives at my office. Beth's skin is pale and warm to the touch. She is in obvious discomfort and slightly bent over. We review her symptoms over the last twenty-four hours, and it appears she is experiencing some sort of gastrointestinal disorder, perhaps a stomach or intestinal virus.

Before the exam, my nurse informs me Beth has a low-grade fever of 100 degrees. Beth is obviously afraid, but a sonogram shows everything is fine with her baby, and she seems to relax somewhat. During the sonogram, Beth flinches as the transducer moves over the right side of her abdomen. I continue with the exam, gently and methodically applying pressure at various places on her abdomen.

Next, I press down on the lower right portion of Beth's abdomen and release the pressure quickly. She flinches with pain, a re-action doctors call *rebound tenderness*. I ask her to straighten her legs, hold them together, and raise them six inches off the table. The action causes her obvious discomfort. My conclusion: Beth has appendicitis.

I call a talented general surgeon with whom I went to medical school and explain my findings. He agrees to meet Beth at the hospital and take over her care.

I explain Beth's diagnosis to her and tell her what to expect once she arrives at the hospital. I also notify the obstetrician covering my practice that night about what is happening. Beth's husband arrives and takes her to the hospital. As they leave, they promise to call me day or night if they have any questions or concerns, and return the following Friday for a checkup.

There is no further word from Beth until she returns one week later for her follow-up appointment. Her recounting of the chain of events that occurred the preceding week leave me aghast.

When Beth was admitted to the hospital, she was immediately given IV fluids, and her blood work was sent to the lab. She was given medication for her nausea and started to feel somewhat better. Her white blood cell count, a marker for infection, was slightly elevated. The surgeon saw her a few hours after admission, but rather than take her to the operating room, he elected to watch her overnight.

By morning, after receiving a large amount of IV fluids and a few more doses of nausea medication, Beth was feeling much better. Her temperature remained below 100 degrees, and an ultrasound performed the night before failed to confirm appendicitis. With this information, the surgeon sent her home.

Now, in my office, Beth is feeling somewhat better, but obviously still not up to par. On examination, the tenderness remains in the lower right part of her abdomen, and the rebound is still present. Beth detects my concern and disapproval of the way the surgeon handled her care. To put it mildly, I am disappointed he did not perform an appendectomy the prior week, and I am not pleased that Beth let a week go by without contacting me.

Still certain she has appendicitis, I explain to Beth that if her appendix ruptures, it could threaten the well-being of both her and her baby. The appendix must be removed immediately. Because of the size of her uterus, the incision will have to be made higher on her abdomen than with a normal appendectomy. Anesthesia is safe, and the incision alone will do nothing to disrupt her pregnancy. I send Beth to the hospital to be prepped for surgery.

While waiting to get into the operating room, I call the general surgeon to tell him we are going to surgery immediately. To my dismay, he still insists Beth doesn't have appendicitis.

In the operating room, I make the incision well above the top of Beth's uterus. I enter the abdomen easily and identify the appendix without manipulating the uterus. It is swollen, inflamed and densely matted to the ovary. Although I have done a number of appendectomies in my life, this one makes me extremely nervous. Even the slightest mistake could cause Beth's bowel contents to spill into her abdomen – a life-threatening condition for mother and baby. For this reason, I call on the general surgeon to perform the procedure.

He arrives quickly and skillfully removes the appendix, without any intestinal spillage. Upon examination of the removed appendix, the surgeon flippantly declares, "It's an appendiceal (a herniation in the wall of the appendix) and not appendicitis. That is why I was fooled."

But the final pathology proves I was right to be concerned. It reveals acute and chronic appendicitis.

The following morning, Beth appears to be a different person. Although she is uncomfortable from the surgery, the pain and ill feeling she was experiencing earlier are now gone. I perform another bedside ultrasound, with reassuring results. Beth's baby is moving around, oblivious to the occurrences of the past twenty-four hours.

Beth recovers very quickly, and when I see her two weeks later, she gives me a huge hug and a peck on the cheek. Beth trusted me, and I trusted my instincts, with positive results.

Four months later, I happily deliver Max, her healthy infant son.

CHAPTER 26

What Went Wrong and Why

Introduction

Beth's story highlights the number-one reason women find themselves on the operating room table during pregnancy – appendicitis, or inflammation and infection in the appendix. Although pregnancy does not increase the incidence of appendicitis, it's a possibility the obstetrician must always bear in mind when the patient is experiencing abdominal pain. As pregnancy progresses, diagnosing appendicitis becomes more difficult for a number of reasons.

First and foremost, as the uterus grows, it pushes the appendix upward and outward. As this happens, the symptoms of appendicitis change. The pain associated with this condition is usually less severe than in a woman who is not pregnant; nausea and vomiting are variable; and fever is usually low-grade or absent. Further, although the white blood cell count may be elevated, this symptom also occurs during normal pregnancy.

The two most reliable findings for diagnosing appendicitis in a pregnant woman are abdominal rebound and tenderness during rectal exam. Diagnostic tools that are typically helpful, such as ultrasound and CT scan, are less reliable during pregnancy. Moreover, a CT scan should be avoided if at all possible during the first and second trimesters due to radiation exposure concerns for the developing fetus.

Dr. E. A. Babler was entirely correct when he stated in 1908, "The mortality of appendicitis is the mortality of delay."

This chapter explores relationships – between physician and patient, between physician and consultant, and between covering obstetricians. By now, you may have noticed a continuing theme throughout this book centering on open, effective communication. Maintaining good communication, and recognizing and intervening when it breaks down, are the best ways to ensure your pregnancy ends safely and positively.

This chapter also covers surgical situations that may arise during pregnancy, the signs and symptoms to watch for, diagnostic tests, and treatment options. Although these circumstances are uncommon, when they do arise, prompt diagnosis and therapy are the keys to ensuring a healthy outcome for you and your baby.

Facilitating Communication

Beth was fortunate that appendicitis can fester for a few weeks before actual rupture occurs. Having heard nothing after I sent her to the hospital the first time, I assumed (you know what they say about assuming) she underwent an appendectomy that Friday and everything had gone well. Knowing I would see her in a few days, I spoke with neither my partner, who was on call that night, nor the general surgeon, who assumed her care. This lack of communication was a mistake on all our parts and could have resulted in a tragedy. Thankfully, it did not.

Further, Beth did not contact me. I routinely gave all my patients my cell phone and pager numbers, a practice disdained by virtually all my associates for fear of numerous bothersome phone calls over minor matters.

When Beth's husband took her to the hospital that Friday, I instructed them to call me with any questions or concerns whatsoever. They thought she was going to the hospital to have her appendix removed. That did not happen. After being hydrated by volumes of IV fluids and receiving multiple doses of anti-nausea medication, Beth felt somewhat better. Like most patients, she assumed the surgeon knew what he was doing and, frankly, she was greatly relieved to hear she didn't need surgery. It's easy to understand why she didn't call me.

Both the physician and the patient are responsible for facilitating communication. Clearly, I should have followed up with the general surgeon, my partner or Beth. I probably also should have made it clear she should call if she did not have the appendectomy. Any time health care providers disagree upon a plan of treatment, alarms should go off that something is awry.

As a patient, you need to be proactive and gather all the information possible from all sides to help guide your medical care. When medical professionals disagree, good communication is the mainstay of avoiding potential harm. Never be afraid to question your doctor, even when they have spoken with the consultant. Likewise, don't hesitate to question the consulting doctor. If you are still not clear about circumstances, ask for a meeting of all providers involved.

The Art of Medicine
Diagnostic medical equipment has improved dramatically over the past half-century. Non-invasive techniques such as ultrasound, CT scan and MRI give crystal-clear pictures of different parts of the human anatomy. However, they are not infallible.

Obtaining a complete patient history and asking probing questions are still integral to diagnosing an illness. Combined with a thorough physical exam, these techniques are irreplaceable. Unfortunately, many physicians today rely more on the diagnostic tools available through radiology than on the basics of a good history and physical exam.

Pay close attention to your encounters with your physician. A good doctor asks follow-up questions when given information by the patient, rather than moving quickly to the next category, and puts the patient at ease, rather than rushing them through the visit. The physical exam is thorough, not cursory. The doctor takes time to listen to your heart and lungs, check your thyroid, and perform thorough breast and abdominal exams.

A thorough physician is a physician you can likely trust. Some details you mention may seem inconsequential to you, but they could be very important in reaching an accurate diagnosis. To make that diagnosis, the physician must be attentive. There is a saying in medicine that rings very true: "You can't find a fever if you don't take the temperature." A thorough physical exam often yields subtle, important findings that may be easily missed if the exam is only cursory.

All too often, patients take choosing an obstetrician too lightly. Fortunately, most pregnancies are uncomplicated, with no troublesome events. But when something does go wrong, having the wrong obstetrician puts you and your baby at risk.

Knowing Beth and having a past relationship with her, combined with the subtle findings in her physical exam, helped me make a correct diagnosis and get her to the operating room before disaster occurred.

Avoid Making a Mistake

Many obstetrical offices today have numerous providers, and you may become a patient of the practice, rather than a patient of one of the obstetricians in the group. In such a case, you may feel it is important to see every physician who might deliver your baby. That's not necessarily a good idea. The downside is that that you will not develop a relationship with any particular physician, and no single doctor will truly know you and your pregnancy. That's how mistakes are made. It's highly likely the notes in your chart are the only communication that will ever take place among these practitioners about your care. And a chart is not always read.

Lab results may go unnoticed for a while. Ultrasound reports may not be thoroughly read. Important facts in your past medical history may be overlooked. Future tests one provider feels are important may not be ordered by another.

As the patient, you must *know* your pregnancy. Having one primary obstetrician allows you to do this. Discuss with this physician the things that are important for a covering doctor to know about your medical history and pregnancy. Learn these salient points, and be sure to communicate them to any health care provider you see, other than your primary OB, especially if you are seen at a hospital. Don't be intimidated. They want to know.

To help with this, at thirty-two weeks, you should ask for a copy of your medical record. You can never be absolutely sure at which hospital you will land. You don't need the entire record; most doctors can give you a three- to four-page summary. Be sure your lab and ultrasound summary sheets are included, along with a list of any problems or potential problems with your pregnancy. Remember to keep it with you at all times, especially when traveling.

Be proactive. There are no stupid questions when it comes to pregnancy. When you ask a question, be sure you receive a satisfactory answer that you fully understand. Don't be intimidated, and don't be brushed off. If you have real concerns, they must be addressed to your complete satisfaction. Your body undergoes many changes during pregnancy, and these changes will cause signs and symptoms that will be unfamiliar to you. There is a physiological explanation for each of them. When you question a health care provider about one of these symptoms, you should not accept an answer such as, "That's just normal for pregnancy." Be sure to query exactly what is causing you to have the symptoms you are experiencing.

CHAPTER 27

What Expectant Mothers Should Know About Surgery and Pregnancy Conditions Requiring Surgical Intervention

Introduction

When faced with the prospect of surgery while pregnant, your obvious first reaction is, "How will this affect my baby?" In twenty years of practice, I don't recall any mother ever asking about her own safety before first asking that question. Obviously, the maternal instinct begins at conception.

Fortunately, almost any surgical procedure can be performed without putting your baby in jeopardy. This is true as long as your medical team follows all the proper steps. That requires effective communication and close collaboration among your obstetrician, anesthesiologist, consultants, and nurses.

A number of considerations must be addressed prior to surgery. Knowing these issues and ensuring they will be handled properly will help maximize the chances of a safe outcome for your baby.

Anesthesia

Virtually all anesthetic agents will cross the placenta and reach your baby to some degree. The main exception to this is a category of medications called *muscle relaxants*, which are used to paralyze the muscles during surgery. This is one of the reasons general anesthesia is safe during pregnancy.

The other reason anesthetics are safe during pregnancy is the unique fetal circulatory system. The anatomy of the fetal heart and major blood vessels differs dramatically from those of a human living outside the uterus. That is because, while still in the uterus, your baby gets its oxygen from your blood, not via its own lungs. Various openings in your baby's heart and great vessels exist only while the baby is in your uterus. The effect of these openings is to shunt the majority of the blood your baby receives to the lower part of its body. Therefore, only about 10 percent of this blood reaches your baby's brain.

Many studies have looked at the effects of general anesthesia and fetal anomalies. Virtually every study has found no connection. One or two of them found a possible relationship between anesthetic exposure and neural tube (brain and spinal cord) defects at a very early gestational age of about four to five weeks. If at all possible, general anesthesia should be avoided during this period. If unavoidable, ultrasound and blood studies at fifteen to twenty weeks can determine whether your baby was affected.

Regional anesthesia, spinals and epidurals are covered in another chapter of this book. The largest risk associated with these anesthetics is a drop in your blood pressure, causing your baby's heart rate to decrease. If these anesthetics are used, your blood pressure must be monitored and treated aggressively, and if at all possible, the fetus should also be monitored.

Diagnostic Studies

Doctors rarely declare a surgical emergency without first performing diagnostic procedures. At a minimum, your obstetrician will order blood work to help with diagnosis. The two most common evaluations are white blood cell count and hematocrit. An elevated white cell count can indicate infection, and a decreased hematocrit can indicate internal bleeding.

Typically, radiological studies are the most concerning. The connection between radiation exposure and fetal defects is well-known to mothers. It is less well-known that fetal defects resulting from radiation exposure depend entirely on the dose and the baby's gestational age. A single x-ray will have no effect on your baby, regardless of gestational age. Thousands of studies have looked at this issue and concluded any dose under 5 rads is insignificant to your baby's well-being. In fact, there is support in medical literature to suggest any dose under 10 rads is safe.

A chest x-ray taken from two views exposes your baby to only one-hundredth of one rad of radiation. Ideally, you should avoid any radiation exposure, but if it's necessary, ask the radiologist what the total dosage of radiation will be for the test being performed.

The risk of fetal injury from a properly administered diagnostic procedure that involves some fetal radiation exposure is negligible, at most, other than between eight and twenty-five weeks of gestation. The greatest risk occurs between eight and fifteen weeks. Between fifteen and twenty-five weeks, a much higher radiation dose, usually greater than 50 rads, is required to cause injury.

Other than fetal defects, the concern with radiation exposure is an increased risk of cancer. The actual risks for prenatal exposure are unknown; however, from data accumulated from atomic bomb survivors, it would appear that there is virtually no increased risk with under five rads of exposure. Above five rads the risk increases in very small percentages with increasing doses. Over a lifetime, it is estimated that prenatal exposure to fifty rads would increase your baby's risk of cancer over the general population by as much as approximately 15 percent. Although that may sound frightening, remember that a chest X-ray with two views involves exposure to only one-hundredth of one rad.

A number of diagnostic modalities use no radiation at all. Magnetic resonance imaging (MRI) gives a picture somewhat similar to a CT scan; however, MRI uses magnetic fields, rather than ionizing radiation, and is entirely safe during pregnancy. Ultrasound uses sound waves and is also completely safe.

As with any medical procedure, you must weigh the risks of a diagnostic procedure involving radiation versus its potential benefit to you and your baby. Should the need for diagnostic testing arise, discuss this in detail with your obstetrician and radiologist.

Surgical Considerations

There are a number of factors to consider prior to undergoing surgery, and the timing of the surgery is high on the list. The safest time to perform surgery is during your second trimester. Although most surgeries involve emergencies, when timing is beyond your control, surgery can be postponed in some instances until you reach the second trimester. Another important consideration is choosing a procedure that minimizes uterine manipulation and exposure to irritants, thereby greatly reducing your chance of going into preterm labor. No matter what your surgical emergency, these two considerations must be at the forefront of your obstetrician's mind.

Other than manipulation, the three main irritants to be concerned about are blood, pus, and powder. Some surgical gloves are coated in powder, although not nearly as often as they used to be. Confirm with your surgeon that all surgical gloves used will be powder-free. If this is not possible, request all surgical personnel rinse their gloves in sterile water prior to starting the procedure.

Free pus in the abdomen portends a dismal prognosis for your baby's survival. That is why surgical intervention for an inflammatory condition like appendicitis should be done sooner, rather than later. When performed early enough, most surgical procedures involve very little risk for your pregnancy. If a wait-and-see approach is taken, you should be hospitalized with very close monitoring to avoid the terrible complications that accompany rupture of an inflamed organ.

Blood is also a tremendous irritant to the uterus. For this reason, you should discuss with your surgeon steps that can be taken to minimize blood exposure in the abdomen. For instance, a vertical skin incision causes much less blood loss then a transverse one. Moreover, a laparoscopic procedure should involve virtually no blood loss at all. The ability of the surgeon to clearly see the operative site, called *exposure*, is a key factor in minimizing complications. This can be accomplished either laparoscopically, or through the correct size and location of an abdominal incision. This should be dictated by the kind of surgery planned and the size of your uterus.

Beth's case is a perfect example. Normally, when performing an appendectomy, a small, angled incision is made in the lower-right side of the pelvis. Because of the size of Beth's uterus, and to minimize blood loss and maximize exposure, I chose a vertical incision above her naval. Once I saw the size and inflammatory response surrounding her appendicitis, I actually enlarged the incision to get better exposure. By doing this, I decreased the amount of blood lost and minimized the chances of rupturing the appendix while trying to remove it.

Laparoscopy should only be attempted if you are less than twenty-two to twenty-four weeks' gestation, and only if your surgeon is an experienced laparoscopist. When laparoscopy can be safely performed it has many advantages over open surgical techniques. The incisions are much smaller, recovery time is much shorter, blood loss should be minimal, and visualization of the operative site is usually much better.

When a laparoscopy is performed, the abdominal cavity is usually filled with carbon dioxide, which raises the anterior abdominal wall up and away from the rest of the organs, allowing visualization of the entire abdominal contents using a telescope-like instrument. When laparoscopy is used on a patient who is not pregnant, pressures of up to twenty millimeters of mercury (mmHg) of carbon dioxide can be used, increasing visualization. When used on a pregnant woman, the ideal pressure is ten mmHg and absolutely should not surpass fifteen mmHg. This is because the mother will absorb some of the carbon dioxide, which can lower her pH and potentially cause problems with the baby. Fortunately, the anesthesiologist is able to measure your carbon dioxide levels, allowing the surgeon to operate safely.

Without a doubt, the prospect of undergoing surgery while pregnant is frightening, but when it is performed in a timely manner with proper incisions, there should be no negative consequences for your pregnancy.

Fetal Monitoring During Surgery

The degree of fetal monitoring that is appropriate during surgery depends entirely on your baby's gestational age. If your baby is previable (less than twenty-four weeks), continuous monitoring during surgery is not performed. Your obstetrician or a labor-and-delivery nurse will check your baby's heart rate immediately before surgery and again in the recovery room.

If your surgery is being performed after twenty-four weeks, ideally, continuous fetal monitoring during the procedure should be elected. This is accomplished with either an external fetal monitor or an ultrasound machine. Both can be covered with a sterile plastic drape to prevent contamination of the operative field. The kind of surgery you have and the placement of the incisions will dictate the modalities to be used.

If ultrasound is chosen, it can be performed either through the abdomen or through the vagina. Monitoring is usually intermittent, rather than continuous.

The neonatal team should also be consulted prior to surgery. If an emergency delivery is necessary, they can respond quickly with appropriate equipment. If at all possible, the surgery should be performed in an obstetrical operating room to enable the neonatal team quicker access, if needed.

Finally, monitoring for preterm labor is also an integral part of your care. This monitoring does not take place during surgery, but should occur in the recovery room immediately afterward. With the exception of progesterone, medications to stop contractions typically are not given prior to surgery.

If you are experiencing contractions after surgery, this is usually due to uterine irritability, not preterm labor. Terbutaline or magnesium sulfate, the medications of choice to stop preterm labor, will almost always stop these contractions.

Conditions Requiring Surgical Intervention

Generally, pregnancy does not increase your risk of needing surgery. The two exceptions to this rule are cervical incompetence and gallbladder disease.

The cervix bridges the uterus and vagina. It is mostly made up of connective tissue, and remains closed and firm until the end of pregnancy. However, in some women, the connective tissue is not strong enough to hold the baby inside, and the cervix begins to dilate painlessly. If no intervention is taken, the baby is delivered prematurely. Certain risk factors, such as multiple dilation and curettages (D&Cs), can put you at risk for this condition. By taking a thorough history, your obstetrician is usually able to determine whether any risk exists.

If you are at risk, you will be followed with multiple pelvic exams and/or serial ultrasounds. If surgery is required, it is usually only a five-minute procedure, performed vaginally under light anesthesia, in which a purse-string suture is placed at the junction of the top of the cervix and the lower part of the uterus. This is very effective in preventing preterm delivery, especially if performed between twelve and fifteen weeks.

High levels of progesterone, produced by the placenta during pregnancy, decrease the contractility of smooth muscle. This is what puts you at risk for constipation and gallbladder-related symptoms.

Because the gallbladder does not empty as efficiently during pregnancy as at other times in your life, pregnancy may slightly increase your risk of gallstones or inflammation. Fortunately, gallbladder disease is usually not life-threatening and can be treated medically, without surgical intervention.

Should surgery become necessary, this is one situation in which laparoscopy would probably be the preferred method. The gallbladder is located in the upper-right quadrant of the abdomen beneath the rib cage. Because of this location, the uterus is rarely an impediment to laparoscopic access. This surgery is performed by a general surgeon, not an obstetrician.

Other conditions that may require surgery include intestinal obstruction, breast cancer, ovarian tumors or cysts, and kidney stones. Although these are the most common indications during pregnancy, any illness that may require surgery in the non-pregnant state could also require surgery while you are pregnant.

CHAPTER 28

Questions to Ask Your Doctor

The prospect of surgery is never pleasant, and it can be frightening when you're pregnant. Try to remain calm and have a family member present for all consultations with your doctors, if possible. Two surgical scenarios may present themselves – an acute emergency and a non-emergent condition that can be resolved electively.

The most important question applies only if your pregnancy is past twenty-four weeks: can the hospital care for your baby, if emergency delivery is necessary? If at all possible, be sure it can, and that the neonatal team is not only aware of the surgery, but on standby in case they are needed.

Acute

- What kind of incision will your doctor make, and is it the best one to minimize uterine manipulation?

- How will the baby and uterine activity be monitored before, during, and after surgery?

- Who will perform the surgery, and what is the surgeon's level of experience?

- If an obstetrician will not perform the surgery, will one be present to oversee the surgery and ensure minimal manipulation of the uterus? (The answer should be "yes.")

- What possible effects will the different medications being used during surgery have on my unborn child?

- Are you sure surgery is absolutely necessary now? What are the possible consequences to me and my baby of having a period of observation? Can any other tests be performed to help shed light on the diagnosis?

Elective
- All but the last question listed above apply here as well. In addition, the following questions apply when the surgery can be done electively.

- When is the safest time to perform the surgery and why?

- What are the possible consequences of not having the surgery at all?

- Are you sure of the diagnosis? Are there any further tests that may help clarify the issue?

- What is the safest form of anesthesia?

Although potentially very worrisome, when handled appropriately, most surgeries during pregnancy can be performed safely and with very little risk to your baby. Many conditions that require surgery during pregnancy have the potential to cause peritonitis (infection throughout your abdominal cavity) if left untreated. This is far more dangerous to both you and your baby than surgery itself, and steps to prevent this from occurring (i.e., not delaying the surgical procedure) should be taken.

Finally, if time allows and you are wary, never be afraid to ask for a second opinion. This could come from a surgeon, an obstetrician, a high-risk obstetrician, or another specialist knowledgeable about your condition.

PART IX

Electronic Fetal Monitoring Interpretation During Labor and Delivery

CHAPTER 29

An Electronic Fetal Monitoring Primer

A basic understanding of fetal monitoring is paramount to ensuring your baby's safe travel through the labor and delivery process. As we previously explained, your baby communicates with the outside world through fetal monitoring tracings, which are graphs of your baby's heart rate printed on strips of paper. These tracings are extremely useful measures of how your unborn child is withstanding changes in environment and stimuli during the birthing process. Fetal monitoring tracings (sometimes referred to as *fetal monitoring strips*) give doctors and nurses a real-time, overall picture of your baby's condition throughout labor. While the paper strips are printed out in your room, monitors in various locations throughout the labor and delivery suite also display your baby's tracings in real time.

There are several brands of fetal heart rate monitors, but they are all similar in design and work on the same principles. The monitor gives both auditory and visual feedback about your baby's heart rate, and records the frequency and duration of your contractions. Information about the fetal heart rate appears on the upper portion of the paper, and information about your contractions is seen at the bottom.

Fetal heart rate tracings are interpreted by analyzing several features of the heart rate pattern called *baseline, variability, accelerations,* and *decelerations.* These features, particularly decelerations, are not analyzed in a vacuum. Understanding the relationship between changes in your baby's heart rate and your uterine contractions – specifically, when those changes occur in relation to your contractions – is essential to fetal heart rate monitoring.

Characteristics of the Fetal Heart Rate Patterns

The baseline heart rate of a fetus is determined by observing the fetal heart rate over a ten-minute period. The heart rate must remain relatively stable (within a range of up to five beats per minute) for at least two minutes. We say *relatively* stable because, to a certain degree, variations in fetal heart rate from beat to beat and minute to minute are expected. Typically, the rate per minute at which the heart beats for the majority of time during a period of relative stability is rounded to the nearest five-beats-per-minute figure, such as 120 or 125. That rounded figure is referred to as the *baseline* heart rate. Baselines are sometimes described less precisely, such as *in the 120s.*

A normal baseline fetal heart rate ranges between 110-160 beats per minute. During labor, fluctuations in baseline within these parameters are expected, but downward changes must be differentiated from *prolonged decelerations,* as defined below.

Variability refers to the changes in your baby's heart rate from beat to beat and minute to minute. A baby's heart rate should not remain static, which would present as a flat line. Instead, your baby's heart rate should appear as a saw-tooth pattern. Another important factor is the degree of variability, which is characterized as follows:

- Absent variability = amplitude range undetectable;

- Minimal variability = fewer than six beats per minute;

- Moderate variability = six to twenty-five beats per minute; and

- Marked variability = more than twenty-five beats per minute.

With absent variability, no saw-tooth pattern whatsoever appears on the tracing; instead, the pattern appears as a relatively flat line. This circumstance is always of concern, but even more so if it exists for longer than ten minutes. Minimal or marked variability lasting more than thirty minutes also must be addressed by your health care providers.

Once the baseline is established, when reviewing succeeding tracings, you may see periods of fifteen seconds to a couple of minutes when the baby's heart rate is fifteen to twenty-five beats or more above the baseline. These elevations in heart rate signal fetal movement and are known as *accelerations*. Just as your heart rate increases when you exercise, your baby's heart rate increases with movement. The presence of accelerations is very reassuring that your baby is adequately withstanding the rigors of labor.

You also may also notice on EFM tracings periods during which your baby's heart rate drops below the baseline. These are called *decelerations*. There are three types of decelerations – *early*, *late* and *variable*. These names are derived from the relationship of the decelerations to your contractions.

An early deceleration is believed to be caused by compression of your baby's head as it descends in the birth canal. It begins during the onset of the contraction and ends before the contraction subsides. As noted above, the data about the fetal heart rate appears on the top portion of the EFM strip, and the data about your contractions is seen at the bottom. The shape of the baby's heart rate deceleration, as traced on the strip, should mirror the shape of your contraction. If it does, you should not be concerned about this type of deceleration.

A variable deceleration may or may not be associated with a contraction and can appear anywhere on the EFM strip. Caused by compression of the umbilical cord, this type of deceleration appears on the tracing in a shape that appears similar to the letter "V" because the baby's heart rate drops quickly and recovers quickly. Variable decelerations are usually not concerning, but can be problematic at times and may even require intervention.

A drop of thirty beats per minute is not uncommon with a variable deceleration; however, if it involves any of the following characteristics, you should raise concern and demand immediate attention:

- Occurs with every contraction over a period of fifteen to twenty minutes;

- Consistently drops below eighty beats per minute over a ten- to twenty-minute time period;

- Lasts more than fifty to sixty seconds, and constitutes a drop in heart rate greater than sixty beats per minute from the baseline or a drop below eighty beats per minute, irrespective of the "baseline" (tracing on the EFM strip appears wide and deep);

- Loses variability (the saw tooth pattern in the heart rate tracing flattens out); or

- Repeatedly does not return to baseline until after the contraction has concluded (while the downward angle of deceleration continues to resemble the downward angle of the letter "V," the angle of the upward slant of the deceleration widens out before it returns to baseline).

A late deceleration usually begins during the second half of a contraction and does not end until after the contraction is over. Like early decelerations, the shape typically mirrors the shape of the mother's contraction. They can be subtle – just a few beats per minute below the baseline – or much more obvious, at ten to fifteen beats per minute below the baseline. The most important factor in determining whether you are, in fact, experiencing a late deceleration is the heart rate. If it does not return to baseline until after the contraction is over, it is a late deceleration.

Late decelerations occur because of utero-placental insufficiency. This means too little blood, oxygen and nutrients are getting through the placenta to the baby, and too little of the harmful byproducts in the baby's blood are being cleared through the placenta. This type of deceleration is never good, especially if it becomes repetitive, occurring with more than 50 percent of the mother's contractions.

Measures Available to Improve Fetal Heart Rate Patterns
If any of these concerning patterns occur, they may be corrected by intrauterine resuscitative measures (IURM), which include:

- Repositioning you to either your left or right side;

- Administering oxygen to you;

- Increasing your IV fluids via a large influx of fluid at one time (called a *bolus*);

- Discontinuing Pitocin (a drug used to stimulate the uterus);

- Administering terbutaline (a drug used to relax the uterus);

- Placing a catheter inside the uterus to introduce more fluid (amnioinfusion); and

- Provided your water has broken, placing an electrode on your baby's head to confirm whether the heart rate abnormalities are, in fact, real.

Nurses often institute some of these IURM in the absence of the physician. However, if anything other than a position change is necessary, insist a doctor be called to your bedside and remain there for at least ten to fifteen minutes to assess your status and that of your baby.

If these measures fail to restore your baby's heart to a normal pattern within five to ten minutes, a physician's immediate presence is mandatory. Ask to be moved to the operating room sooner, rather than later. This way, precious time will be saved if a normal fetal heart rate pattern doesn't return and an emergency C-section needs to be performed. No harm will be done if your baby's heart rate pattern returns to normal and emergency delivery is not required. However, please refer to Part IV, Alexandra's Story, which addresses concerns raised and action required if IURMs provide only temporary relief and need to be repeated frequently.

Pay particular attention to the procedures being performed. Stopping the Pitocin and administering oxygen require a doctor's presence immediately. Also, watch the demeanor of the nurses and residents caring for you. If they seem worried, you should be worried. Don't be afraid to question them. Don't be afraid to ask for your doctor or their supervisor. Your baby's health and safety are at stake, so stand up for your child. Studying the EFM strip for longer than thirty seconds, summoning someone else to look at the strip, or asking you to change positions quickly are all signs of anxiety or uncertainty on their part.

Impact of Uterine Contractions

Probably the most important part of understanding the fetal monitor tracing is recognizing and making sense of the contraction pattern and fetal heart rate variability.

The uterus is a muscle. When it contracts, it significantly decreases or cuts off the amount of blood and oxygen your baby receives. This poses no problem under normal circumstances, as your baby has reserves and is able to tolerate this condition. Think of it like holding your breath under water – as long as you stay under no longer than thirty to sixty seconds at a time and take breaths in between, you can keep re-submerging for a long period of time. However, if you stay under longer than sixty seconds and take shorter breaths in between, you will tire quickly. Some of you will tire more quickly than others, but everyone will tire eventually. Babies are no different.

If your contractions last more than one minute or come too close together (more than five in a ten-minute period), your baby will tire over time, and vital organs may be deprived of oxygen, leading to irreversible damage.

What Certain Fetal Heart Rate Patterns Look Like on EFM Tracings

Following are images of various EFM heart rate patterns that you can use to compare with those that appear on your baby's strips. The notations have been added for your benefit. They did not appear and would not appear on a tracing produced by an electronic fetal monitor.

In this tracing (FIG. 3) there are two accelerations (each is at least fifteen beats above baseline, and lasts a minimum of fifteen seconds). The hallmark of moderate variability, a saw tooth pattern of the fetal heart rate tracing, is present. For the most part, the heart rate varies

REACTIVE (FIG. 3)

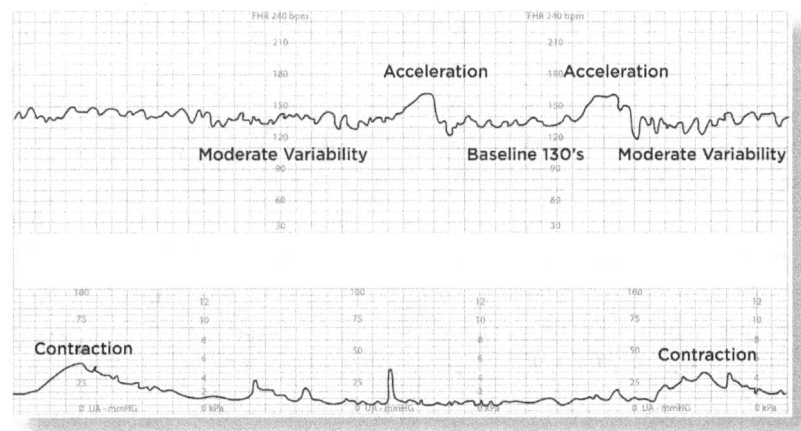

EARLY DECELERATION (FIG. 4)

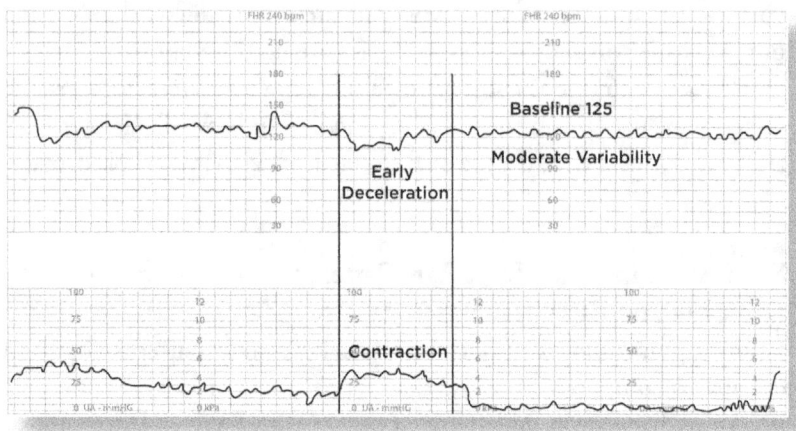

between 130 and 140 bpm, giving us a baseline in the 130's. Most likely, a nurse would document the baseline to be 135 bpm. This tracing is consistent with a well-oxygenated fetus.

This EFM tracing (FIG. 4) exhibits a classic early deceleration, which is caused by pressure being exerted on the baby's head as it travels down through the mother's pelvis. Characteristically, this deceleration begins during the first half of the contraction, and ends before the contraction is completely over. The baseline fetal heart rate depicted is about 125 bpm. Moderate variability of between five and twenty-five bpm is also present. This presentation is very reassuring of a well-oxygenated fetus.

On the following page, the variability is moderate in this tracing (FIG. 5), with a baseline of 150 bpm. A number of variable decelerations are present and identified. Notice how they occur somewhat randomly and differ in the depth that they drop below the baseline. They also go down quickly, and return to baseline quickly, giving the appearance of the letter "V." The decelerations fall in a range from fifteen to thirty beats below baseline. At this point, there is no

MILD VARIABLE DECELERATION (FIG. 5)

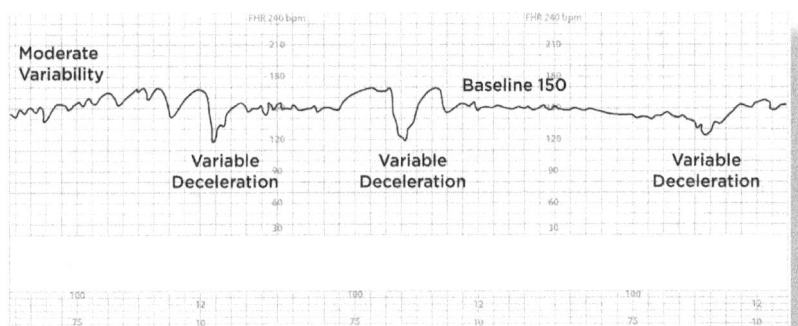

concern of a baby being compromised. When mild variable decelerations appear, often, a position change alone will sufficiently improve the flow of oxygenated blood to the fetus and cause the decelerations to disappear.

This fetal monitor strip (FIG. 6) shows classic late decelerations, which start after the peak of the contraction and return to baseline of

LATE DECELERATION (FIG. 6)

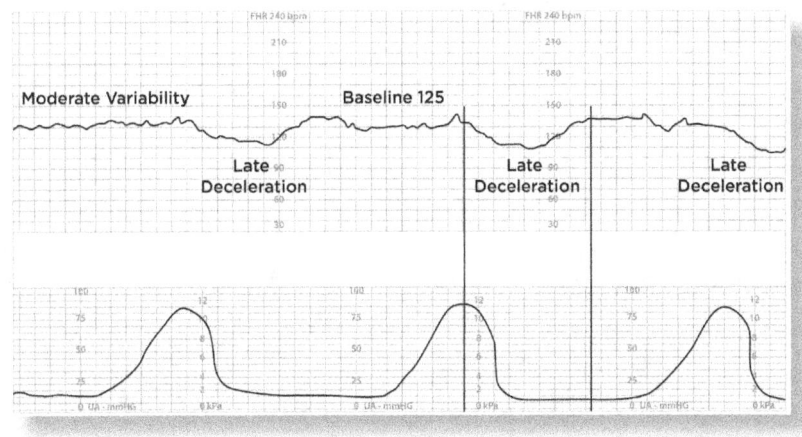

about125-130 bpm after the contraction is over. They occur with each contraction. This degree of repetition signals that the fetus may not be receiving an optimal amount of oxygen. This expectant mother was undergoing labor induction with Pitocin. She had an intrauterine pressure catheter in place, allowing the obstetrical team to assess the strength of the contractions. The contraction pattern, which appears on the bottom half of the strip, reveals the contractions are long-lasting and very strong, and therefore, very stressful on the baby and the most likely cause of the repetitive late decelerations. However, the saw tooth pattern of the fetal heart rate is still present, a positive sign indicating the baby has not exhausted all its oxygen reserves. The obstetrical team realized that they needed to take action to alleviate the added stress. IURM that consisted of turning off the Pitocin, increasing the amount of IV fluids this expectant mother was receiving, and repositioning her onto her left side were effective. The corrective measures quickly improved the flow of oxygen being delivered to this fetus, resulting in the appearance of much improved and reassuring EFM tracings.

Notice the almost complete loss of variability, with nothing left but a trace of the saw tooth pattern (FIG. 7). The baseline is easily

IMMEDIATE INTERVENTION REQUIRED (FIG. 7)

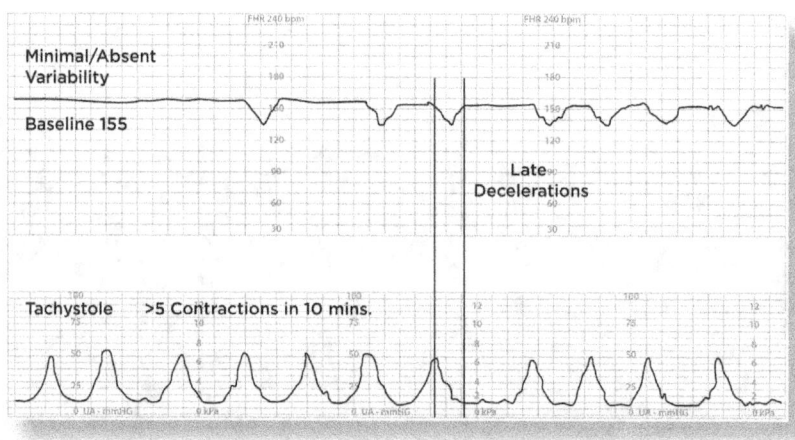

detectable at 155 bpm, and remains there without variation. Each deceleration begins towards the middle of a contraction, and ends after the contraction concludes (consistent with a classic late deceleration). Although the decelerations are initially spaced out, they quickly begin to occur more frequently. When late decelerations occur with more than 50 percent of the contractions, as they do toward the end of this strip, fetal compromise is potentially imminent. This development demands administration of immediate and full IURM. If a reassuring EFM pattern does not return within five to ten minutes, immediate delivery is required.

Fetal heart rate variability is absent in this tracing (FIG. 8). Additionally, the baseline rises with each contraction, and is extremely tachycardic. This is a sign the baby has exhausted all oxygen reserves. The variable decelerations become longer and deeper with each contraction. This is a further indication that no reserves remain. Five minutes later in this strip, the baby's heart rate plummets to fifty and does not recover. An emergency C-section was

LIKELY TOO LATE TO PREVENT INJURY (FIG. 8)

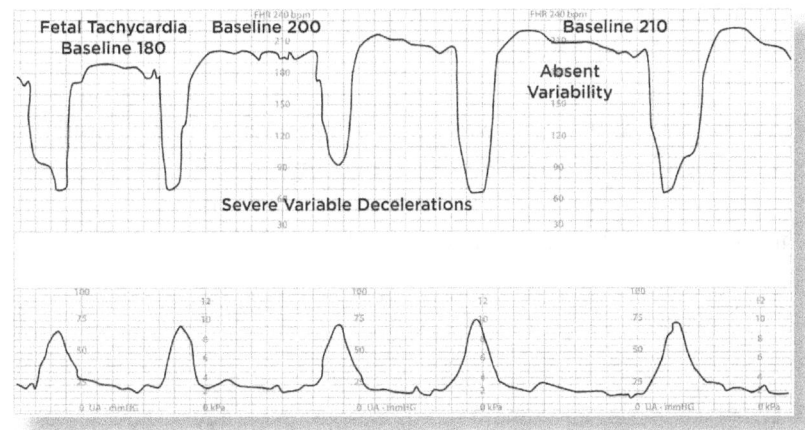

performed. This baby was extremely stressed and unfortunately suffered permanent brain injury.

More About Variability of Fetal Heart Rate

Two things that can affect variability, but are not concerning, are a baby's sleep cycle and certain medications.

Babies' need sleep, just as we do. Typically, they sleep for twenty to forty minutes every few hours. During this time, there is often minimal variability in their heart rate; however, this should last no longer than forty minutes at a time. Likewise, stimulation, as in a pelvic exam, should increase your baby's heart rate.

The narcotics commonly given for pain control early in labor may also affect the appearance of your baby's heart rate pattern. The pattern may exhibit minimal variability, which is an expected side effect. Just as the medication causes you to sleep, it has the same effect on your baby. These changes usually are present during the twenty- to thirty-minute period following administration and then disappear. One caution: if your baby's variability is already diminished, you should try to avoid narcotics, as they can confuse the picture about what is really occurring with your baby.

You Can Do It

Learning the differences between normal and abnormal fetal heart rate patterns mostly involves visual remembrance, not definitions. Learn the normal pattern, and question anything that deviates from it. You can do it. Your health care providers should be grateful to have another pair of eyes watching over your baby.

PART X

Key Points Summary and Birthing Plan

Key Points Summary

Year-in and year-out in hospitals across the United States, normal, healthy pregnancies take a terrible turn during labor and delivery, culminating with the birth of a brain-injured child. Although most birth injuries result from circumstances beyond anyone's control, many others are preventable.

By now, you have read our real-life stories about pregnancies, many of which ended with heartbreakingly bad outcomes. Each bad-outcome case involves significant errors committed by physicians or nurses. These errors were completely avoidable.

The simple truth: The more knowledgeable parents – not just mothers – are about preventable medical errors, the more likely those errors can be prevented or the repercussions from them diminished. The same holds true for anyone playing a supporting role for an expectant mother, particularly once she is hospitalized. During labor-and-delivery someone in a supporting role is in a better position than the mother to buttonhole hospital personnel and facilitate action.

The summary that follows is intended to serve as an abbreviated source of information regarding many of the topics we have addressed.

Selecting a Physician and Hospital

Be sure to ask how often your OB is in the hospital and who covers for your OB when they are not available. Call or visit the website of your state medical board – the state agency that licenses, regulates and disciplines doctors – and check the records of both your primary obstetrician and the backup physician. Another source to consider checking is Healthgrades.com.

Choose a hospital with a twenty-four-hour, in-house anesthesia team. If you decide to use a midwife, make sure your labor and delivery will take place in a hospital, not a birthing center, so you will have immediate access to an operating room if an emergency C-section is necessary.

Prenatal Tests

Be sure your doctor reviews any and all lab results in detail with you at the next appointment after blood has been drawn.

We strongly recommend requesting a herpes blood test with your first set of labs. Many people carry the herpes virus without knowing it, and steps can be taken to ensure your baby's safety, if you happen to be one of them. Although the chance of passing herpes to your baby is small, if it happens, the effects on the baby can be devastating, including possible permanent brain damage.

An ultrasound should be conducted during the second trimester to evaluate your baby's organs, but not before eighteen to twenty weeks. By that time, the fetal anatomy will be clear enough to ensure normal structural development. Afterward, be sure to go through the report thoroughly with your doctor.

First and Second Trimester

You should expect to see your doctor every four to six weeks until you are twenty-eight weeks pregnant. At that point, your visits should become increasingly more frequent – every three weeks, then every two weeks and, finally, once a week for the last three to four weeks.

You should begin to feel your baby move at fifteen to eighteen weeks.

At twenty-four to twenty-eight weeks, all moms should be tested for diabetes because the placenta produces a substance that can affect how glucose is metabolized.

Know your blood type. If you are Rh-negative, have the baby's father tested. If he is Rh-positive, you should receive an intramuscular injection of RhoGAM at twenty-eight weeks. This injection should be repeated immediately after delivery if your baby is also Rh-positive. Failure to receive the second injection could pose a risk to your un-born children in future pregnancies, so nag until you get it.

Unusual pain and/or bleeding, unusual pressure, or abnormal vaginal discharge at any time during pregnancy should always be brought to your doctor's attention immediately.

If you go out of town, take a copy of your patient chart in case you experience any complications. This will ensure the health care providers caring for you have accurate information.

Between OB visits, write down all your questions and concerns, so you remember them when you see your doctor.

During the Third Trimester

Moms are routinely tested at thirty-two to thirty-six weeks for group B strep bacteria, which is the primary cause of meningitis in newborns. This condition is not treated until right before delivery. If you test positive, make sure you receive intravenous antibiotics during labor.

If you notice any decrease in your baby's activity during the last three months of pregnancy, contact your doctor immediately. You may be advised to eat something sweet and lie on your left side, and your baby's movement may quickly return to normal after doing so. If it does not return within one hour, call back immediately. Insist

(FIG. 9)

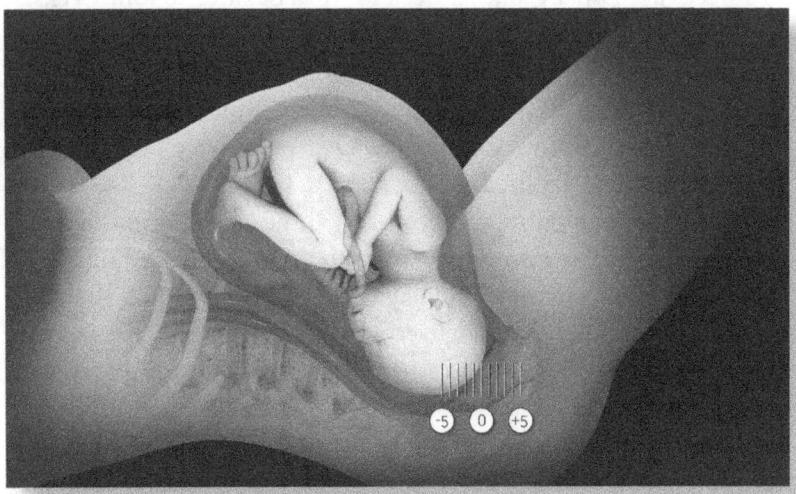

on going to the hospital and having your baby placed on a fetal heart monitor.

If you have not delivered by forty-one weeks, weekly testing should be performed to confirm the placenta is still functioning properly and your baby is receiving adequate oxygen and nutrients. Ideally, you should not pass forty-one and a half weeks without delivering. If your cervix is not favorable for induction by this time, delivery by C-section should be seriously considered, especially if your baby's head is not close to engagement.

This picture (FIG. 9) illustrates a baby in the vertex (head-down) position at approximately zero station. The fetal station is the measurement of the distance of the lead part of your baby's head (related in centimeters) from the ischial spines. The ischial spines are bony prominences that can be felt on either side of the vaginal wall. Station is determined during vaginal exam by your health care provider, who locates the spines and then estimates the distance of your baby's head above or below them. When the head is located exactly at the spines it is called zero station (at this position the fetal head is now engaged in your pelvis). Positions above the spines range from -1 to -5, and positions below the spines range from +1 to +5. Once your baby is crowning, it has reached +5 station.

If you develop medical issues during the third trimester that warrant fetal monitoring, and you are told you may need to be induced due to worrisome fetal testing, you should seriously consider demanding a C-section. Prior to making this decision, you should have a thorough discussion with your doctor about the exact nature of the concern, anticipated time to delivery after induction, potential risks of induction, and how quickly a C-section can be performed if problems arise during induction. This discussion should be documented on a consent form that both you and your doctor sign. Do not risk the health of your unborn baby over a misplaced belief that one form of delivery is better than another.

Hospital Admission for Normal Delivery
Make a note of the time you arrive at the hospital for delivery. A delay of thirty minutes to an hour before getting you into a labor room is fine, but any longer is unacceptable because the baby needs to be on a fetal heart monitor.

In Labor and Delivery
You should expect that continuous electronic fetal heart rate monitoring will be performed in order to aid in the assessment of your baby's well-being. External electronic monitoring uses an ultrasound transducer to listen to the fetal heart rate through your abdomen. The sounds of the fetal heart are then transmitted to a computer, with the pattern ultimately being displayed on a monitor, and printed on a roll of graph paper.

Your movement, your baby's movement and other factors such as obesity may make it difficult to adequately track your baby's heart rate using external monitoring. If a problem reliably monitoring your baby's heart rate externally develops and it cannot be quickly rectified, you should insist that your OB switch to internal EFM as soon as possible. The factors listed above that may interfere with external monitoring don't ordinarily interfere with internal monitoring. Remember, however, internal monitoring involves attaching an electrode directly to your baby's scalp, which cannot be done until your cervical and membrane status allow.

Internal monitoring should also be employed as soon as possible following the presence of either recurring abnormal fetal heart rate patterns, or an abnormal pattern that cannot be timely corrected by IURM. Indeed, internal monitoring should be resorted to whenever closer monitoring than external monitoring permits is appropriate.

Once you are in the labor-and-delivery suite, if there are concerns about your baby's heart rate pattern, you should insist on seeing a doctor immediately.

If Pitocin is administered, be aware it can affect your baby's heart rate and oxygen supply. Preferably, a laboring mother on Pitocin should be on an internal pressure catheter to monitor the strength, frequency and duration of contractions. You should not have more than five contractions every ten minutes, and they should last no longer than sixty to ninety seconds each, with at least a full minute of rest in between. If your contraction pattern is not within these limits, the Pitocin could be hyper-stimulating your uterus, which could adversely affect your baby. Time the contractions and alert your nurses to excess contractions. You should also insist on seeing your OB if you are experiencing any unrelenting pain or a burning sensation in your abdomen. If there is any delay, speak to the nurse manager without delay.

Whenever shifts change or a nurse or doctor provides a second look at or opinion about your baby's tracings, it is important to get the big picture, and not just the way things look at the moment. Under these circumstances, a review of the tracings over the previous hour or longer provides a more reliable picture.

While you shouldn't feel compelled to constantly watch your baby's EFM tracings, don't be shy about taking a good look every now and then, particularly following implementation of IURM. You may want to keep this book handy so you can refer to the examples of normal and abnormal fetal heart rate patterns. Do not exclusively rely on your own interpretation. Rather, use your knowledge to ask questions and help you decide whether to request that another pair or two of trained eyes, particularly those of a nurse supervisor (known as a *charge nurse*) or your OB, take a close look at your baby's heart rate pattern. In any event, if your nurse puts you on oxygen or places you on your left side, that's an indication she is concerned about something, and you should be, too. If IURM don't produce a normal fetal heart rate pattern or even if they do, but they only provide temporary relief and must be reinstituted, insist on seeing a physician immediately. Do not accept any delay.

Have the nurse explain the EFM strip to you, and then watch the fetal heart monitor. A baby's baseline heart rate will vary between 110 and 160 beats per minute. It is normal for it to dip below the baseline rate for a few seconds, but a drop of greater than five beats in the heart rate for more than three minutes is a matter of concern, especially if the drops form a recurring pattern. If this is the case, insist a doctor be called to come to the bedside immediately.

If your baby is in trouble, it is critical for the hospital to be prepared to perform an immediate C-section. In a true emergency, every minute counts. In some circumstances, a uterine rupture, for example, a delay of only a few minutes can have very serious consequences. It is better to have the doctor and delivery team ready and available, and not need them, than for an unnecessary delay to cause your baby to suffer lack of oxygen and be born with permanent brain injury as a result.

Use of forceps or a vacuum carries risks for your baby. If your baby is younger than thirty-five or thirty-six weeks, a vacuum should never be used. Further, neither a vacuum nor forceps should be used unless the baby is at the +2 station position or greater. If this becomes an issue, request an immediate C-section. If the request is refused, document your request and get hospital personnel to sign it. While some laboring mothers may feel a C-section is somehow a failure on their part, that is simply not the case, and it is far better than exposing your baby to undue risk of injury.

Epidurals can affect your blood pressure and, therefore, your baby's heart rate. Prior to receiving an epidural, it is imperative that you quickly be given one liter of intravenous fluids (known as a *bolus*) to help decrease the possibility of adverse effects. After the epidural is placed, fetal monitoring is critical. Around 10 percent of babies will experience a slowing of the heart rate due to the epidural. Most recover fairly quickly, but if the drop extends past three to five minutes, insist on being transferred to the operating room immediately. Once there, the baby's heart rate should be re-checked. If it has returned to normal, it is safe for you to continue laboring; however, if it is still down, a C-section should be performed immediately.

If you are being given an epidural for an elective C-section, the baby should be monitored from immediately after the epidural placement until the surgery is ready to begin.

Spinals are commonly used for anesthesia during C-sections. They have the same effect as epidurals, only much more quickly. It is imperative the surgery be performed immediately after placement of the spinal, so be sure the operative team is ready to begin. The doctors should be in the OR, scrubbed and gowned, prior to the placement of the spinal. If there is to be any delay, insist on fetal monitoring until the surgery begins.

Both spinals and epidurals are safe forms of anesthesia, as long as the hospital staff takes the proper precautions to monitor your baby's well-being.

Laboring mothers should always have an IV inserted, even for normal deliveries and even if no fluids are expected to be needed. This helps avoid losing precious minutes in case an emergency arises and medication or anesthesia is required.

If you elect to use a midwife, make sure:

- Continuous fetal heart monitoring is used;

- A backup physician is assigned;

- You will labor in the hospital, not a birthing center;

- You know where the physician is located, and how long it will take them to reach the hospital; and

- You meet the backup physician.

Using a Birthing Plan to Set the Parameters of the Labor-and-Delivery Care You Expect to Receive

A birthing plan is an informal written contract between the hospital, your physician and you. It should be a comprehensive account of both yours and your partner's expectations of how you will interact with your doctors, nurses and other hospital personnel during labor and delivery.

We strongly suggest that you have an aggressive, proactive birthing plan in place. You should carefully review your final birthing plan with your obstetrician or midwife. Ask that they sign it, place a copy in your prenatal chart, and send a copy to the hospital. Initially, they may be unreceptive, but if you are firm in communicating your plan's importance to you, most will abandon their hesitation. However, if they continue to object, you should seriously consider choosing a different provider.

Our birthing plan is distinctive from those you will find in other books written for expectant parents. They tend to recommend subjects to be discussed, but leave you to make decisions without guidance. Further, they seemingly instruct you to let the doctor control all important decisions. For instance, the authors of *What to Expect When You're Expecting*® suggest your "request should be tempered by what the other side [your OB] finds acceptable."

We believe your instructions should be followed and your requests honored so long as they are reasonable and time permits. You shouldn't feel as though you must compromise or accede to the doctor's preference about a course of treatment unless there are no reasonable alternatives. On the other hand, compromising or giving in on issues that don't involve protecting the well-being of you or your baby, such as the number of visitors in the delivery room, is often the right thing to do.

We contemplate a new direction for health care in which the patient plays a primary role. You cannot be deemed to have given "informed consent" if your doctor has done nothing more than hold your hand and reassure you things will be fine. To truly give informed consent, you must have had an intelligent discussion with your doctor about the benefits and risks of proceeding with a given plan, the alternatives, and the physician's experience and comfort level with each. All risks commonly associated with each potential procedure should be discussed in detail until you are satisfied you have a good understanding on which to base a decision.

Your baby's safety comes first, and settling for the minimum standard of care will not ensure it. While some of the suggestions in our proposed birthing plan are controversial, in our opinion, they are the safest course to a healthy outcome for you and your baby.

Birthing Plan

My Expectations During Labor and Delivery

You can download this plan with places for your partner, doctor and you to sign at MyAdvocates.com/Secrets.

1. I will be settled in a labor-and-delivery room, and my unborn baby will be connected to a fetal heart monitor within one hour of arriving at the hospital for a routine delivery.

2. Once in the labor-and-delivery suite, I will be seen by a physician immediately if I experience unrelenting pain (continuous pain without relief between contractions), significant vaginal bleeding, or my baby's heartbeat cannot be detected.

3. An IV will be inserted and ready, even if no fluids are expected to be needed.

4. If my baby's fetal heart rate pattern cannot be reliably assessed by external electronic fetal heart monitoring, an internal monitor will be substituted as soon as my cervical and membrane status permit. Furthermore, internal monitoring will be employed as soon as possible if my baby develops a recurring or prolonged abnormal fetal heart rate pattern, or intrauterine resuscitative measures (IURM) are required and are not effective within ten minutes. In addition, if internal monitoring is employed for any of these reasons, I will be seen by a physician without delay.

5. If I am given Pitocin, an intrauterine pressure catheter will be employed as soon as possible after my cervix has dilated enough to allow its placement, and my water has broken.

6. If the baby's heart rate drops more than five beats below baseline for three minutes or longer, a physician will be called immediately to provide bedside management. If my baby's heart rate falls more than five beats below baseline for more than five minutes, I will be moved immediately to the operating room. Once there, the baby's heart rate will be checked again, and if signs of impending fetal harm are still present, an immediate C-section will be performed.

7. My first priority is the health and safety of my baby. If my baby requires IURM and the fetal heart rate does not become reassuring within ten minutes, irrespective of whether monitoring is being accomplished externally or internally, I will be informed, and my physician will be notified immediately and will see me without delay.

8. I will be consulted prior to the use of a vacuum or forceps. This consult will include the reason for their use, a discussion of the progress of my labor, the current location and orientation of my baby's head in my pelvis, realistic chances of success, and any inherent risks specific to my situation. Should I decide to have a C-section instead, this decision will be respected.

9. My baby will be monitored after the placement of an epidural. If an epidural or spinal is being used for a C-section, my baby will be monitored until surgery commences.

10. A pediatric team will be available in the delivery room to resuscitate my baby, if there is meconium present in my amniotic

fluid, or if there is any reason to suspect that at birth my baby may have an abnormally low heart or respiratory rate.

11. Any concerns my family or I may have will be addressed professionally and patiently, using layman's terms.

In our opinion, this proposed birthing plan is reasonable and provides a course for safe delivery. You may wish to use all or some of our suggestions in your plan, and you may add conditions specific to your pregnancy or requirements that are important to you, personally.

However, sometimes during labor, the best-laid plan must be set aside. That is particularly true when a life-saving emergency develops, such as uterine rupture or massive hemorrhaging resulting from abruption or placenta previa. Under emergency circumstances such as these, trust your health care providers' experience and skill. This is not a time to lose precious minutes in negotiation.

Finally, always keep a copy of your birthing plan with you. When you arrive at the hospital, you will have it available in case the hospital or covering physician did not receive it. If this is the case, review it with them, and ask them to sign it and place it in your medical chart.

Postpartum

Although we are not pediatricians, we believe a few words of caution are in order to warn you about potential issues to watch for in your baby.

In a number of cases, our clients' newborns went home from the hospital with undiagnosed infections that were allowed to continue through the first several weeks of life, leading to meningitis and permanent brain injury.

You have read about the group B strep test pregnant women undergo between thirty-four and thirty-six weeks of gestation. Unfortunately, just because you test negative at that time does not mean you won't test positive at the time of delivery. If your baby contracts this bacteria and it is not treated in a timely manner, the results are devastating. To complicate matters, group B strep can attack within twenty-four to thirty-six hours after delivery or even later, between seven and fourteen days of life.

If you have a fever during labor and delivery, you should have a heightened awareness of your baby's condition during the first two weeks after delivery. Your instincts about your baby's health are always paramount, but they are especially crucial with respect to watching for signs of group B strep. As little as a six-hour delay in getting antibiotics can mean the difference between a complete cure versus a permanent brain injury.

If your baby has contracted group B strep, the early symptoms will be subtle. However, they can progress very quickly to full-blown seizures – an indication it is too late. The early signs to look for in your baby are:

- Decreased or no interest in feeding;

- Less activity or longer periods of sleeping;

- Difficulty arousing the baby from sleep;

- Changes in bowel movement pattern, color or consistency;

- Little or no urine output in the diaper; and

- A low-grade fever or even more concerning temperature instability (inability to maintain a normal temperature).

Your baby may have one or more of these symptoms and not have group B strep, but the danger is too great to take any chances. If you have any concerns whatsoever, call your pediatrician immediately and make sure your baby is seen that same day. If your doctor cannot accommodate you, go to the emergency room.

New mothers are often perceived as overly worrisome and not taken seriously. Do not accept this attitude. You must insist your baby is tested. If you had a temperature during delivery, were group B strep-positive, or your membranes were ruptured for more than twelve hours, this is important information to give your providers.

At minimum, insist that your baby's blood is tested. These tests should include a complete blood count (CBC) with a differential to include a count of the number of bands present, an electrolyte panel and a C-reactive protein (CRP) analysis. The most important tests are the band count and the CRP. If they are normal, it is unlikely an infection is present. If they are abnormal, even slightly, blood cultures should be performed and antibiotics started until the culture results return. Alternatively, these tests can be repeated six to eight hours later to look for trending patterns.

If you are sent home, your baby is probably fine and should begin to improve over the next twenty-four hours. However, if your baby's condition seems to be worsening, don't hesitate to return to the doctor or hospital for reevaluation.

Remember to be on the lookout for the signs and symptoms listed above during the first thirty-six hours of life, and then for the first few weeks of your baby's life.

Herpes can be an equally devastating pathogen, but because it is a virus, it is more difficult to cure. Typically, it strikes between ten and twenty-one days of life. This is why we recommend all women be tested for the virus during their initial prenatal visit. If you tested negative for herpes, it is extraordinarily unlikely your baby will contract it. If you tested positive, it is imperative to tell your pediatrician and discuss signs to look for in your baby. All the signs, symptoms and remedial steps that applied to group B strep also apply to herpes.

When I became a first-time father, a very wise, seasoned and respected pediatrician told me, "Giles, if your baby is pooping and eating, she is fine. If this changes, call me."

This advice may seem simplistic, but it is right on target. Many, if not most, of the infections and other maladies that your baby can develop reveal themselves, to some degree, in your baby's eating, digesting, eliminating and sleeping habits.

PART XI

GLOSSARY OF OBSTETRICAL TERMS

Note: The definitions in this glossary are stated as they pertain to babies, although many terms apply to adults, as well. For example, arterial blood gas tests are performed on adults, as well as on infants.

abruption. Premature separation of the placenta from the uterine wall.

acceleration. An increase in the fetal heart rate of fifteen or more beats above the baseline lasting fifteen seconds or more from the beginning of the increase until the return to baseline. In a baby less than or equal to thirty-two weeks gestation, the fifteen by fifteen changes to ten beats by ten seconds. Any of these increases that last ten minutes or more are no longer considered accelerations, but rather are a change in baseline.

acidemia. A decrease in the pH of the baby's blood below 7.2.

ACOG – American Congress of Obstetrics and Gynecology.

amniocentesis. A test in which a long needle is inserted through the mother's abdomen and uterus, into the amniotic cavity, to remove amniotic fluid for genetic or other fetal testing, or possibly to decrease an excess volume of amniotic fluid.

amniotic cavity. The space inside the uterus that is surrounded by membranes and contains amniotic fluid, your baby and the umbilical cord.

amniotic fluid. The fluid surrounding your baby in the womb. It is virtually all water, but also contains salts and fetal cells. It protects the baby, keeps the baby warm, and helps with lung and digestive tract development.

Apgar. A score from zero to ten assigned to babies at one and five minutes of life to reflect their well-being. Five categories are assessed, with a maximum of two points assigned to each. The higher the score, the more reassuring your baby's status, with seven or greater considered normal.

Apgar Score

Apgar Numbers	2	1	0
Appearance	Normal color (hands and feet are pink)	Normal pink body color, hands and feet are bluish (acrocyanosis)	Pale or blue all over
Pulse (heart rate)	Normal (above 100 bpm)	Below 100 bmp	Absent (no pulse)
Grimace (reflex irritability)	Pulls away, coughs or cries with stimulation	Facial movement only with stimulation (grimace)	Absent (no response to stimulation)

Activity	Active, flexed arms and legs that resist extension	Arms and legs flexed/some-what flexed	No movement or flexion, "floppy" tone
Respiration (rate and effort)	Normal rate and effort with a good cry	Slow or irregu-lar breathing, grunting and weak cry	Absent (no breathing)

apnea. An episode of not breathing.

arterial blood gas. A test in which blood is drawn from one of your baby's arteries or umbilical artery. This test is conducted to determine the acid-base status and oxygenation of your baby's blood.

AROM – artificial rupture of membranes. A procedure in which a nurse or doctor uses an instrument to break the membranes of the amniotic sac (surrounding your baby and palpable through the cervix) to release amniotic fluid. This is commonly done during labor to speed the process to delivery.

asphyxia. An occurrence in which your baby is deprived of oxygen for a long enough period to cause harm.

augmentation of labor. The use of medication, almost exclusively Pitocin, to increase the strength and frequency of uterine contractions.

auscultation. When a health care provider listens to your baby's heartbeat.

AWHONN – Association of Women's Health, Obstetric and Neonatal Nurses.

baseline FHR – baseline fetal heart rate. The heart rate during a ten-minute period, rounded to the nearest five-beat-per-minute increment, excluding periods of accelerations, decelerations or marked variability. The measurement must be taken for at least two minutes to accurately determine the fetal heart rate baseline.

BP – blood pressure.

bpm – beats per minute.

BPP – biophysical profile. A test usually performed in the third trimester to determine your baby's health while in the uterus. Five categories are measured, one by fetal heart monitoring and four by ultrasonography. Each receives a score of zero or two; the higher the score, the more reassuring your baby's well-being.

BPP Components

Category	Normal (2 points)	Abnormal (0 points)
EFM/FHR/NST	At least 2 accelerations in 20 minutes	Less than 2 accelerations in 20 minutes
Fetal breathing movements	At least 1 episode of rhythmic breathing for more than 30 seconds in 30 minutes	No breathing or an episode of less than 30 seconds in duration
Activity/gross body movements	At least 3 movements of the torso or limbs	Less than 3 movements

Muscle tone	At least 1 episode of active bending and straightening of the limb or trunk	No movements or movements that are slow and incomplete
Amniotic fluid	At least 1 vertical pocket greater than 2 cm. in the vertical axis	Largest vertical pocket less than or equal to 2 cm.

brachial plexus. A series of nerves that control movement and feeling in the shoulder, arm and hand.

bradycardia. A condition in which the fetal baseline heart rate decreases below 110 beats per minute.

breech. A circumstance in which your baby's feet or buttocks enter the birth canal first, rather than the baby's head.

CBC – complete blood count. A test that measures different cells in your blood to identify anemia, leukemia, infection, and clotting disorders related to platelet count.

cerclage. A suture placed around the cervix at the internal os (opening) to treat an incompetent cervix, which is a weak cervix that may open too early in pregnancy, resulting in premature birth.

Cervidil. A medication delivered by a vaginal insert used to start cervical effacement and dilation. The insert is placed at the back of the vagina.

cervix. The lowest part of the uterus, connecting the uterine cavity to the vagina. The cervix is usually three to five centimeters in length prior to the onset of labor. The opening to the uterine cavity is called the *internal os*, and the opening to the vagina is called the *external os*.

chorioamniotitis. Inflammation of the placental membranes, usually caused by infection.

chromosomes. Proteins found in the nucleus of cells that carry genetic identities.

CMV – cytomegalovirus. A member of the herpes family, commonly transmitted by toddlers.

corkscrew maneuver. Used in shoulder dystocia, a procedure by which the doctor places a hand against either the anterior or posterior aspect of the baby's shoulder and rotates it in an attempt to dislodge the entrapment.

CP – cerebral palsy. A group of movement disorders frequently associated with problems relating to speech, cognition, epilepsy (seizures), communication, feeding, breathing, and coordination, among others. A significant percentage of cases are caused by preventable medical errors resulting in permanent brain injury.

CPR – cardiopulmonary resuscitation. Various maneuvers, such as chest compressions and positive-pressure ventilation, used to re-establish a heartbeat and respirations.

CRP – c-reactive protein. A blood test used to detect infection.

CST – contraction stress test. A test performed to assess fetal oxygen reserves. During contractions, the amount of blood, and, therefore, oxygen, flowing to the placenta and baby decreases. Contractions are induced using either Pitocin or maternal nipple stimulation. The test, which requires six contractions in twenty minutes, is reassuring when no late decelerations are present. It is non-reassuring if late decelerations occur with greater than 50 percent of the contractions. If neither of these patterns is present, the test is equivocal, and further testing such as an ultrasound exam or biophysical profile may be necessary.

C-section. Caesarean section. A procedure in which the baby is delivered via an incision in the lower abdomen.

CT – computerized tomography scan.

culture. A test of bodily fluids, including but not limited to urine, blood, cervical mucus, and amniotic fluid. The purpose is to detect the presence of bacteria and infection.

CVS – chorionic villus sampling. A sampling of a very small part of the placenta taken toward the end of the first trimester to enable genetic testing of your baby. The placenta is accessed through the cervix, using ultrasound for guidance.

Cytotec. A medication used to start cervical effacement, dilation and labor. It can be taken orally or placed at the back of the vagina.

D&C – dilation and curettage. A surgical procedure performed after a delivery in order to remove uterine contents, such as piece of placenta that was left behind. Removal of products of conception, for instance, during a miscarriage or abortion, is another time this procedure is indicated. It is also used to remove uterine tissue in the non-pregnant woman for diagnostic purposes.

decelerations. A decrease in the baby's heart rate of at least fifteen beats per minute below the baseline fetal heart rate and lasting from thirty seconds to two minutes. A deceleration lasting from two to ten minutes is called a *prolonged deceleration*. A deceleration lasting longer than ten minutes constitutes a change in the baseline fetal heart rate.

dilation. The measurement of the opening of your cervix measured in centimeters. Zero is considered *closed*, and ten is considered *fully dilated*.

Doppler. Also known as a *Doptone*, this hand-held ultrasound device gives a digital readout of the fetal heart rate.

edema. The accumulation of fluid outside the blood vessels, causing swelling. Edema is very common in the feet and ankles near the end of pregnancy.

effacement. The thinning of the cervix.

EFM – electronic fetal monitor.

EFW – estimated fetal weight.

EKG/ECG – electrocardiogram.

EONI – early-onset neonatal infection. Infection in the baby within seventy-two hours of birth.

ephedrine. A medication used to rapidly reverse hypotension.

epidural. An injection into the fatty space surrounding the spinal cord for pain relief during labor and delivery, or before performing a C-section.

episiotomy. An incision from the vagina into the perineum.

Erb's palsy. Injury to the upper nerves in the brachial plexus.

ETT – endotrachael tube. A thin plastic tube inserted through the mouth into the trachea and then attached to one of several devices to assist with breathing via positive-pressure ventilation.

extubate. To remove an endotracheal tube.

failure to progress. A circumstance in which the cervix fails to dilate to ten centimeters, despite adequate labor.

famciclovir/acyclovir. Two variants of medication that are given to mothers with a history of herpes to help prevent transmission of the virus to the baby.

fetal. Pertaining to the baby.

fetal heart monitor strips. The paper recording of the baby's heart rate and mom's contractions.

FHM – fetal heart monitor. Recording your baby's heart rate and pattern on strips of paper. This can be done with an external monitor that is placed on your lower abdomen, or by an internal monitor attached to your baby's scalp.

fifth disease. An infection caused by the parvovirus B-19.

forceps. Similar to salad tongs, these instruments are placed on either side of the baby's head to assist in delivery.

fundal. Refers to the top of the uterus.

GBS – group B strep. A common bacteria found in many women's rectum and vagina, and the number-one cause of neonatal meningitis.

gestation. The time period from the first day of your last menstrual period until your baby's birth.

gestational diabetes. Diabetes present only during pregnancy.

HCP – health care provider.

HCT – hematocrit. The percentage of red blood cells circulating in your blood vessels.

HgB – hemoglobin. The iron-containing protein in the red blood cell. Responsible for oxygen transport to, and carbon dioxide transport away from, the cells in your body. It makes up about 35 percent of the total red blood cell; therefore, the hemoglobin count in a blood sample is typically about one-third the value of the hematocrit.

HSV – herpes simplex virus.

hyperstimulation. An old term for tachysystole, meaning more than five contractions within ten minutes.

hypertonic. A contraction lasting longer than two minutes.

hypotension. A significant drop (usually, 25 to 30 percent or more) in blood pressure.

hypotonic. Lacking muscle tone.

hypoxic. Lacking oxygen.

incompetent cervix. Also know as insufficient cervix, this is a cervix that may not be strong enough to carry a baby to term.

induction. Using medications to start the labor process.

intubate. Place an endotracheal tube into the trachea to assist with breathing.

ischial spines. Bony prominences felt through the vaginal wall at the four o'clock and eight o'clock positions.

IUGR – intrauterine growth restriction. A circumstance in which the baby is smaller than the tenth percentile of babies the same gestational age.

IUPC – intrauterine pressure catheter. A thin, plastic, fluid-filled tube inserted through your cervix, into the uterus, to measure the strength of your contractions.

IURM – intrauterine resuscitative measures. A series of actions taken to increase blood flow and oxygen to your baby.

IV – intravenous.

jaundice. Yellowish pigmentation of the skin sometimes seen in babies after birth.

KB – Kleihauer-Betcke. A test that detects the presence of fetal red blood cells in mom's blood circulation.

Klumpke's palsy. Injury to the lower nerves in the brachial plexus.

labor. Cervical change brought on by uterine contractions. Prior to thirty-seven weeks of gestation, it is called *preterm labor*. There are three stages of labor: (1) the time it takes your cervix to dilate to ten centimeters, (2) the time it takes to push your baby out, and (3) the time it takes to deliver the placenta.

L&D – labor and delivery.

laparoscopy. A minimally invasive surgery utilizing a scope with a camera; long, thin instruments; and very small incisions.

Leopold maneuvers. A series of examinations performed by your health care provider to determine the baby's presentation.

LGA – large for gestational age. A fetus that measures larger than the ninetieth percentile for its gestational age.

L/S – lecithin-sphingomyelin.

macrosomic. Literally meaning *big body*, this term is unrelated to gestational age and is used when a baby weighs more than 4,000 grams (eight pounds, thirteen ounces). In recent years, this number has also been quoted as 4,500 grams (nine pounds, three ounces).

MAS – meconium aspiration syndrome. A condition that occurs when the baby breathes meconium-stained amniotic fluid into its lungs, which can cause serious respiratory and blood pressure issues immediately after birth.

maternal. Pertaining to the mother.

McRobert's maneuver. The flexion of the mother's thighs back onto her abdomen.

meconium. The first bowel movement a baby passes. About 20 percent of the time, this occurs prior to delivery, staining the amniotic fluid a greenish color. This normally does not harm the baby, unless it is breathed it into the lungs.

meningitis. Inflammation of the membranes surrounding the brain, often leading to permanent brain injury.

MFM – maternal fetal medicine specialist. An obstetrician with extra training to manage high-risk pregnancies (also known as a perinatologist).

midwife. Usually (but not always) a nurse, the midwife is trained to perform uncomplicated prenatal care and deliveries.

miscarriage. Unintentional loss of a pregnancy.

MRI – magnetic resonance imaging.

neonatal. The period of time from birth to one month of age.

NICU – neonatal intensive care unit.

nitrazine paper. A yellow paper that turns blue in the presence of amniotic fluid, it is used to test for rupture of membranes.

NST – non-stress test. A test performed with an electronic fetal monitor for twenty minutes. Test results are reassuring when good variability is present and two accelerations occur within that time frame. A reassuring NST is called a *reactive* or *positive NST*. If the test is not positive, the mother is often given a sugar load, and the test is repeated.

oligohydramnios. When the deepest vertical pocket of amniotic fluid is two centimeters or less.

OB – obstetrician. A physician whose practice is limited to pregnancy and childbirth.

OB/GYN – obstetrician and gynecologist. A physician that takes care of pregnant and non-pregnant women.

OR – operating room.

oxytocin. A natural hormone produced in the brain and released from the pituitary gland. One of its important functions is stimulating uterine contractions during labor.

pelvimetry. Evaluation of the maternal bony pelvis for adequate room to enable a safe vaginal delivery.

perinatal. The time of birth or near birth. This term can also refer to the period from twenty weeks of gestational age to one month after birth.

perinatologist. An obstetrician with extra training to manage high-risk pregnancies (also known as a maternal fetal medicine specialist).

perineum. The tissue between the vagina and the rectum.

PG – phosphattidylglycerol.

Pitocin. The synthetic form of the hormone oxytocin, used to induce contractions of the uterus.

placenta. A temporary organ formed during pregnancy that facilitates the transfer of oxygenated blood and nutrients from the mother to the fetus, and deoxygenated blood and waste products from the fetus to the mother.

PPROM – preterm premature rupture of membranes. An occurrence when the amniotic sac breaks prior to thirty-seven weeks of gestation, without contractions.

PPV – positive-pressure ventilation. The provision of air or oxygen under pressure.

presentation. The position of your baby in the uterus.

previa. Abnormal positioning of the placenta at or near the internal opening of the cervix, so all or part of the opening is covered by the placenta.

PROM – premature rupture of membranes. Breach of the amniotic sac in the absence of contractions (prior to one hour before the onset of labor).

pulse oximetry. A non-invasive method of measuring the oxygen saturation of the blood. **quickening**. Mother's first perception of fetal movement.

RBC – red blood cell. One of the values measured in a complete blood count is the red blood cell count, which is a measurement of the total number of red blood cells in your body.

RhoGAM. A medication given to prevent Rh-negative mothers from forming proteins that could attack the red blood cells of the baby's future siblings during future pregnancies if their blood is Rh-positive.

scalp electrode. A small device placed on your baby's head during labor to directly monitor the fetal heart rate.

shoulder dystocia. An occurrence in which one of the baby's shoulders becomes stuck behind the mother's pubic bone during vaginal delivery or, in rare cases, becomes lodged posteriorly in the hollow of the sacrum.

spinal. Injection of an anesthetic agent into the fluid-filled sac surrounding the spinal cord.

station. The distance of the lead part of your baby's head (related in centimeters) from the ischial spines. When the head is exactly at the spines, it is called *zero station*; locations above the spines range from -1 to -5; and positions below the spines range from +1 to +5.

STD – sexually transmitted disease. Some examples include gonorrhea, chlamydia and syphilis.

supra-pubic pressure. Pressure applied at a 45-degree angle to the baby's shoulder just above the maternal pubic bone.

SVE – sterile vaginal exam.

tachycardia. A fetal baseline heart rate above 160 beats per minute.

tachysystole. Also called *uterine hyper-stimulation*, when the mother experiences more than five contractions within a ten-minute period.

terbutaline. Also called *Brethine*, this medication is used to stop or slow uterine contractions.

tocodynomometer. Also called a *toco*, this device is strapped to mom's abdomen (over the top part of the uterus) to determine the frequency, duration and relative strength of contractions.

PART XI

TORCH test. A blood test for toxoplasma, rubella, cytomegalovirus, and herpes.

toxoplasma. A protozoan found in under-cooked meat and in cat feces.

ultrasound. A non-invasive device that uses sound waves to portray a real-time video image of your baby in the uterus. It is also used to guide placement of instruments in amniocentesis and chorionic villus sampling.

umbilical cord. Membranous structure containing blood vessels and extending from the placenta into the baby's umbilicus.

umbilical blood gas. A sample of blood taken from one of the vessels in the umbilical cord to determine the acid-base status of your baby at birth.

umbilicus. Pertaining to your navel (belly button).

vacuum extractor. A suction cup placed on the fetus' head to assist with delivery.

variability. The beat-to-beat changes in your baby's fetal heart rate.

VBAC – vaginal birth after C-section. Often, it is safe to attempt a vaginal delivery, even though you have undergone a prior C-section.

vertex. Presentation in which your baby enters the birth canal head-first.

VZIG – varicella-zoster immune globulin.

PATIENTS' RIGHTS AND DOCTORS' WRONGS®

VZV – varicella-zoster virus. A member of the herpes family, this virus causes chicken pox and shingles.

womb. Another term for uterus.

X chromosome. One of two chromosomes involved in sex determination, XX indicates female gender.

Y chromosome. One of two chromosomes involved in sex determination, XY indicates male gender.

Zavenelli maneuver. A life-saving procedure performed during a severe shoulder dystocia in which the doctor pushes the baby's head back into the vagina and then performs an emergency C-section.

PART XII

About the Authors

HOWARD A. JANET

Making a Difference in Birth Injury and Other Medical Malpractice Litigation

Howard A. Janet, Esq. is recognized as one of the nation's preeminent medical malpractice attorneys, widely known for his aggressive, passionate representation of children who develop cerebral palsy (CP) as a result of preventable birth injuries.

More than 20,000 families have consulted Mr. Janet about potential CP cases. He and his national law firm, Janet Jenner & Suggs, LLC (which includes an in-house, board certified obstetrician-gynecologist), have a proven record of identifying cases in which avoidable medical errors have led to children's CP. When confident a birth injury or other medical malpractice case has merit, Mr. Janet tirelessly seeks the full measure of justice the case demands.

Mr. Janet's tenacity, along with his encyclopedic knowledge and exceptional trial skills, have produced an extraordinary string of precedent-setting results for his clients both in the courtroom and at the settlement table. Representing clients throughout much of the U.S., Mr. Janet and his firm have won hundreds of millions of dollars in verdicts and settlements. But Mr. Janet knows it is not the amount of money he obtains for his clients, especially in birth injury cases, that is the true measure of success. It is what that money can do that makes the real difference – ensure peace of mind and dramatically improve the quality of life for injured children and their families.

Publications and Presentations:

Educating Lawyers, Victims of Medical Errors, and Expectant Parents

Through publications and presentations, Mr. Janet has provided continuing education to attorneys nationwide on the subject of medical malpractice. Writing for Thomson Reuters/Aspatore, he authored the lead chapter of *Inside the Minds: Representing Plaintiffs in Medical Malpractice Cases.* Published in 2013, the book has been characterized as "an authoritative insider's perspective on mounting an effective medical malpractice case." Mr. Janet's presentations include "Birth Injuries and Brain Damage: Legal and Ethical Implications," "Maximizing Your Results in a Medical Malpractice Case," "Settling a Medical Malpractice Case before Suit," and "Wrongful Death." In addition, he served on the National Legal Education Advisory Committee of the American Bar Association program, "The Experts Analyze Brain-Damaged Baby Cases."

As author of *Quick Prep: Navigating a Medical Malpractice Lawsuit – What You Need to Know*, Mr. Janet has helped patients and families harmed by avoidable medical errors become informed consumers of legal services. Published by Thomson Reuters/Aspatore in 2014, *Navigating a Medical Malpractice Lawsuit* has been described as "the ultimate resource for anyone who suspects they have been victimized by medical malpractice."

Encouraging and enabling expectant mothers to take an informed, proactive role in their obstetrical care has been at the forefront of Mr. Janet's literary agenda for ten years. In 2005, *Cerebral Palsy Magazine* published Mr. Janet's article, "The Power of Knowledge: How Electronic Fetal Monitoring Can Prevent Cerebral Palsy." *Patients' Rights and Doctors' Wrongs® – Secrets to a Safer Pregnancy and Childbirth*, co-authored by board certified OB-GYN Giles H. Manley, MD, JD, represents Mr. Janet's latest and most comprehensive effort to help expectant mothers receive the highest quality obstetrical care.

Honors and Awards

The most respected attorney-rating organizations have taken note of Mr. Janet's skills and accomplishments. Martindale-Hubbell® has repeatedly awarded him its highest-possible rating (AV) for legal ability and professional ethics. *The Best Lawyers in America®* and *Super Lawyers®* have consistently identified him as one of the nation's top attorneys. Mr. Janet was honored by *The Best Lawyers in America®* as a "2012 Lawyer of the Year in Personal Injury Litigation – Plaintiffs" and as a "2015 Lawyer of the Year in Product Liability Litigation – Plaintiffs." He is included among the ranks of The National Trial Lawyers® Top 100.

In recognition of extraordinary advocacy in a medical malpractice, invasion of privacy, and sexual abuse class action against the Johns Hopkins Health System (Hopkins), Mr. Janet and a colleague were honored as 2015 Maryland Trial Lawyers of the Year by the Maryland Association for Justice. Mr. Janet and his colleague achieved the largest settlement in U.S. history that involved a single sexual abuse perpetrator. The case stemmed from a Hopkins OB-GYN's use of cameras concealed in pens and other objects to take surreptitious photographs and videos of patients during pelvic exams, and his performance of improper and unnecessary pelvic exams.

Media Recognition of Extraordinary Cases

Mr. Janet has litigated many high-profile cases that have drawn the attention of national media, including *The New York Times*, the

Los Angeles Times, The Wall Street Journal, The Washington Post, Jet Magazine, ABC, CBS, NBC, CNN, ESPN, and news and interview programs such as *Anderson Cooper 360* and *Piers Morgan Tonight.*

Founding a Major Non-Profit Cerebral Palsy Network

Mr. Janet is committed to helping children with cerebral palsy, regardless of the cause. He helped found and provides ongoing support for Cerebral Palsy Family Network (CPFN), a non-profit organization that provides resources and information to families of children diagnosed with CP. CPFN is now the largest Internet-based organization in the world providing support to families touched by cerebral palsy.

Mr. Janet can be reached at HJanet@MyAdvocates.us.

GILES H. MANLEY

BOARD CERTIFIED OBSTETRICIAN-GYNECOLOGIST

Giles H. Manley, MD, JD, is a board certified OB-GYN who early in his twenty-year medical career became convinced that expectant mothers who knew what high quality pregnancy, labor and delivery care looked like were more likely to get the high quality care they deserved. He championed this conviction as he delivered more than 2,000 babies, providing parents-to-be with "insider" information and encouraging them to be proactive in their dealings with health care providers.

Dr. Manley's credentials include certification by The American Board of Obstetrics and Gynecology and designation as a Fellow in The American Congress of Obstetrics. A graduate of the University of Maryland School of Medicine, he received his specialty training at the Greater Baltimore Medical Center (GBMC), including a rotation in high-risk obstetrics at The Johns Hopkins Hospital. A recognized leader in his specialty, he served on both the obstetrical and gynecology advisory committees of GBMC. Later he became Baltimore Area Medical Director and Chief of Obstetrics and Gynecology for health care giant Kaiser Permanente and served on the consortium's regional Obstetrical Quality Review Committee.

A long time and beloved teacher of medical students, Dr. Manley was honored as Teacher of the Year by doctors he mentored in GBMC's residency program – one of his most cherished recognitions.

As Dr. Manley's prominence in his specialty grew, medical malpractice attorneys began seeking his help in analyzing obstetrical malpractice cases. He provided advice and expert testimony for patients' attorneys, as well as attorneys representing doctors and hospitals. In every instance, he "called them like he saw them," providing candid, unbiased opinions.

Becoming a Lawyer to Help Victims of Obstetrical Negligence

Approximately ten years ago, Dr. Manley earned a law degree so he could use his medical and legal expertise to help victims of avoidable obstetrical errors. He is now a highly respected medical malpractice attorney, working hand-in-hand with Howard A. Janet advocating for victims of obstetrical and other medical negligence. Dr. Manley has amassed an impressive record of achieving substantial, much-needed compensation for his clients. In addition, he is the Medical Director of Cerebral Palsy Family Network, the largest Internet-based non-profit organization providing resources and information to families of children diagnosed with cerebral palsy.

Super Lawyers®, an established attorney peer-review publication, recognized Dr. Manley as a "Rising Star" in the field of medical malpractice the first year he was eligible and continues to do so. In addition, he has earned inclusion in the ranks of The National Trial Lawyers® Top 100.

Trial, the journal of the American Association for Justice, has called upon Dr. Manley to use his obstetrical and legal knowledge to help educate fellow medical malpractice lawyers.

Helping Expectant Mothers Obtain the Quality Care They Deserve

Patients' Rights and Doctors' Wrongs® – *Secrets to a Safer Pregnancy and Childbirth* is the culmination of Dr. Manley's efforts to help expectant mothers substantially reduce their risk of falling victim to substandard obstetrical care.

Dr. Manley can be reached at GManley@MyAdvocates.us.

www.ingramcontent.com/pod-product-compliance
Lightning Source LLC
Chambersburg PA
CBHW071031290526
45795CB00004B/1177